LEARN YOGA FOR HEALTH AND WELLBEING

LEARN YOGA FOR HEALTH AND WELLBEING

A gentle week-by-week guide to starting your HOME yoga practice

SUZ STOKES

35 Day Detox Ltd

CONTENTS

This book is dedicated to Rosie,

for providing the inspiration and motivation

to share what I've been teaching in the Kapiti Yoga Studio.

"Calling time on my overthinking and a desire for perfection, plus the ability to laugh at myself, are the greatest gifts of my yoga journey so far."

Suz Stokes

DISCLAIMER

We advise that you check with your medical practitioner before beginning your personal yoga journey. The yoga provided in this book is provided as inspiration, with the intention to show combinations of yoga poses that work together to create a potential outcome. The hope is that you will feel confident to develop your home practice further. However, when doing any physical activity there is a possibility of injury. If you engage in this practice, you do so at your own risk, and agree that 35 Day Detox Ltd and the persons associated with the company have no liability for any injury or loss.

Contact email: suz@35daydetox.com
www.35daydetox.com

Copyright 2024 35 Day Detox Ltd

ISBN PRINT 978-0-473-66703-0
ISBN EPUB   978-0-473-66704-7

First Edition 2024

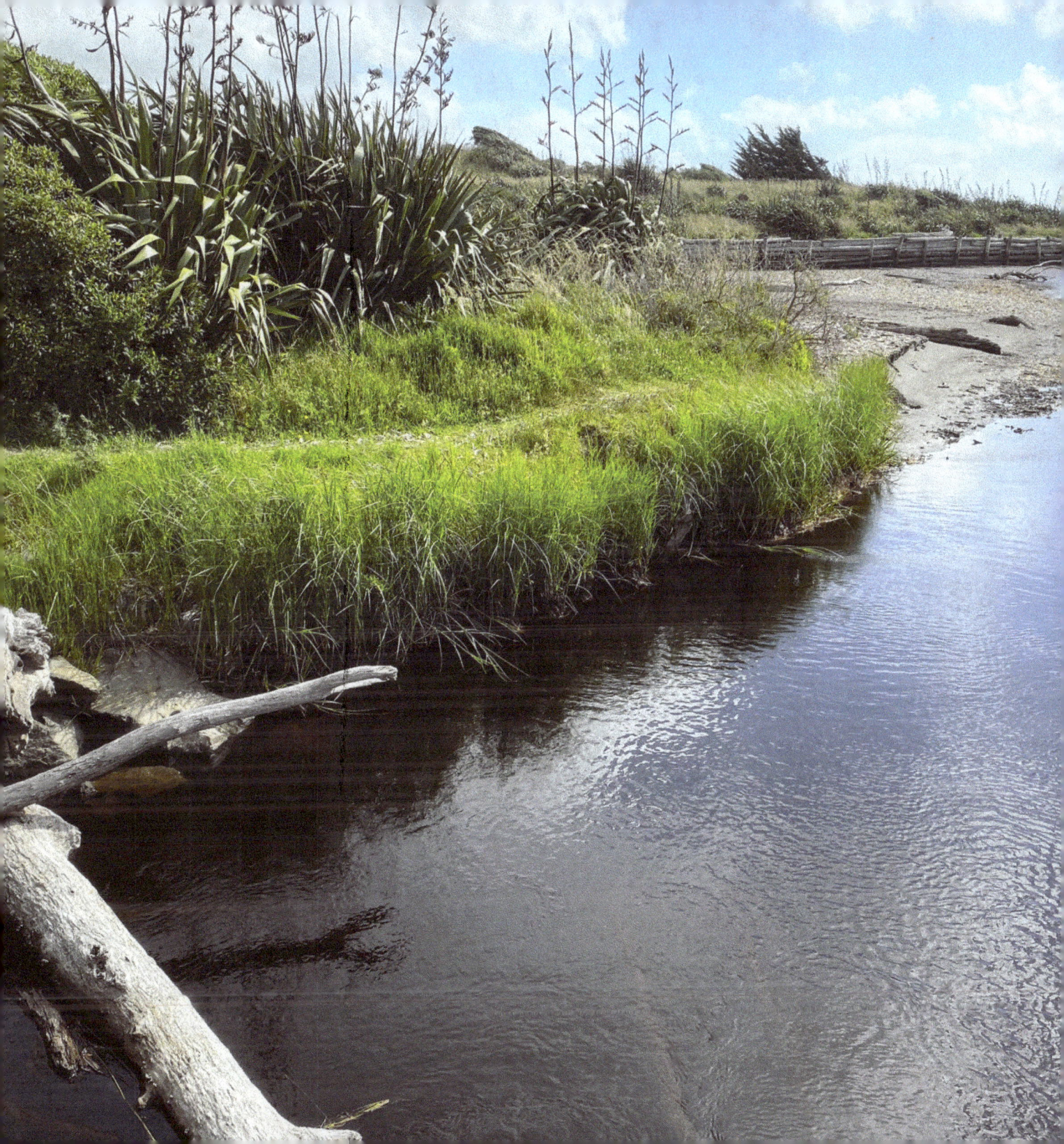

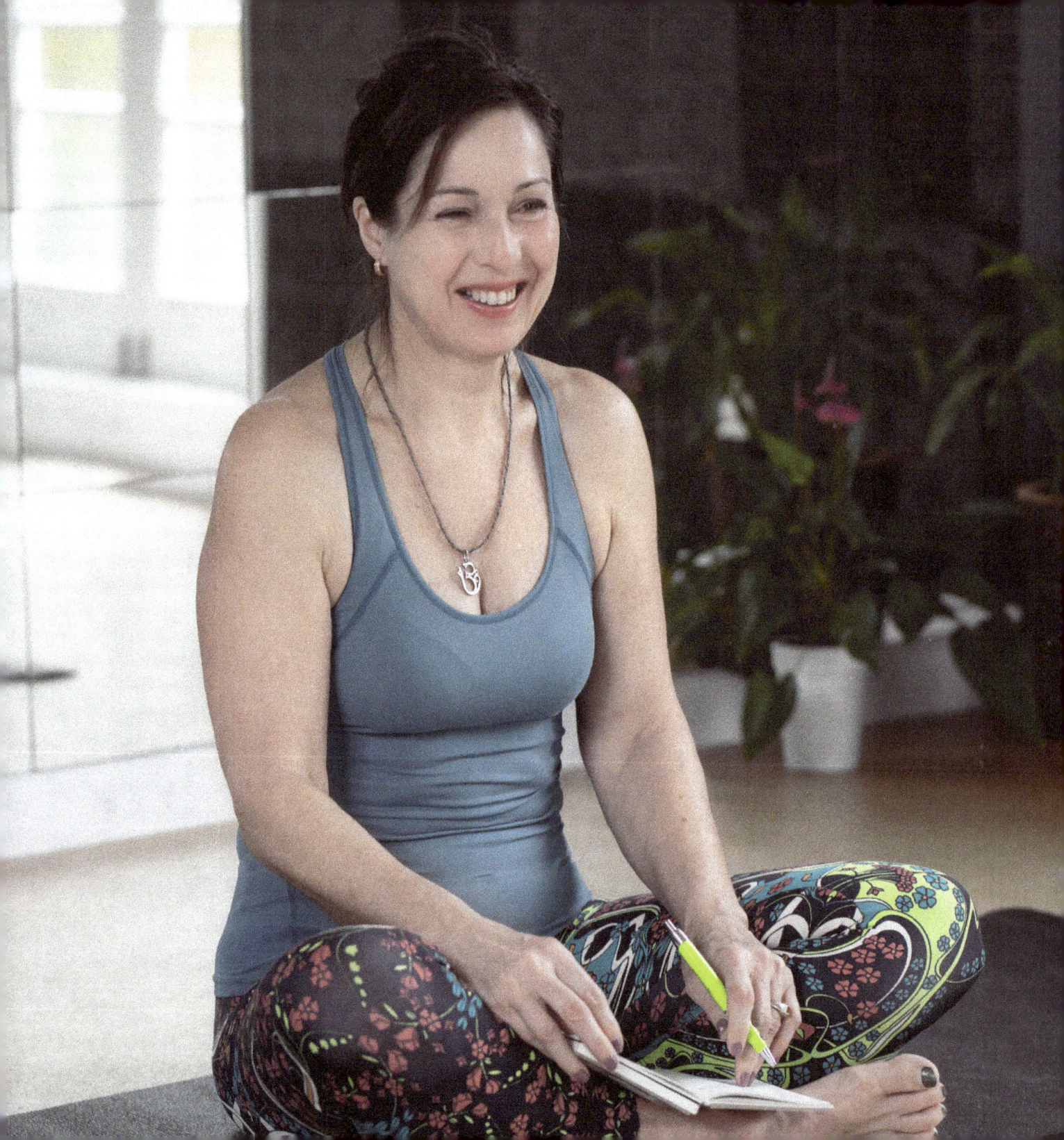

Welcome

Yoga is a powerful tool to have in your kit of self-care. Self-care is never selfish, as prioritising yourself in this way allows you to show up more often in life. Engaging with life can allow you to be of more help to others. Choosing to honour your sense of self, and thereby living an authentic life can make a difference. A regular yoga practice is a very practical, affordable and sustainable way of achieving this!

This program is designed to introduce you to the power of yoga as a daily practice. Your health and wellbeing is the single most important contributor to enjoying life. I think you will agree it is very hard to be calm and happy whilst there are underlying issues of pain. These pains can be physical, emotional and/or mental.

Yoga has been proven to help reduce pain, improve sleep quality, give mental clarity, and deepen your sense of resilience.

By embarking on your personal yoga journey, you are calling time on being held back by physical restrictions and limiting beliefs. You are facing yourself at the present moment and empowering yourself to make the changes you know are needed. One day (on the mat) at a time.

Did you know: The way you show up on the yoga mat is a reflection of the way you show up in life too. We can use this knowledge to decode our patterns, and then we can flip the narrative and use it to manifest change.

YOUR TEACHER AND GUIDE

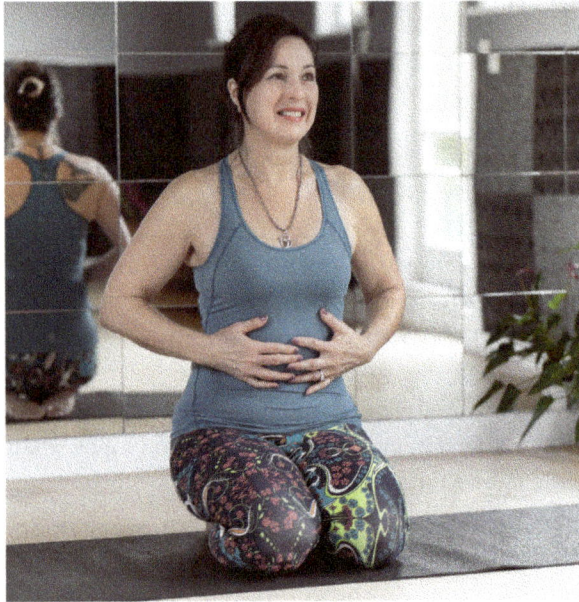

Hi, I'm Suz Stokes and I've been practising yoga and teaching yoga for over 13 years. My belief is that yoga as a personal practice is the perfect way to access improved health and wellbeing.

Not only will it improve your physical presence, it will give you mental clarity and you will radiate peace and harmony. This comes with a very large caveat, because first there are all the aches and pains and accumulated traumas from life's experiences to date, as well as a lot of unprocessed emotions, to be cleared from your body and mind.

I have spent more than 500 hours immersed in learning about (and how to teach) yoga, covering Vinyasa, Hatha, Yin, and Restorative modalities. There is a little bit of each modality in these sessions. I have run a private yoga studio for the past 10 years, specializing in working with individuals to help them improve their health through physical movement and mindfulness.

Above all, I am convinced that yoga is a detoxification process. So much so that in 2014 I founded the 35 Day Detox company. Starting with a desire to share the five week journey of personal transformation, that I knew from experience with myself and my clients, was possible. It evolved to writing a recipe book of healthy foods. In 2021 I chronicled my personal journey of transformation with the book titled "The Physical Manifestation of Self: from High Heels to Yoga Pants with a side of Ironman".

This book has it's beginning in the studio with my private clients - and then became an online program, before heading back to the studio to be taught in a group setting. Throughout those twists and turns the content hasn't changed, giving me confidence to bring it into print now.

GETTING STARTED

In the six weekly sessions of this program you will learn easy yoga poses as well as more challenging options. Take what resonates with you and please leave the rest. It's called "yoga practice" for a reason. You are practicing - not perfect - the main thing is that you show up regularly. Perhaps not every day, but 10 minutes six days a week will be more effective than 60 minutes once a week.

The yoga story goes something like this:

If a farmer wants to find water in the field, then it is better to dig one hole deeply rather than multiple shallow holes. Progress methodically through the program picking a few poses each week that are right for you now. Repeat them until it is time to move on. That way you will get the most benefit from this book and your yoga practice.

Whether you have done yoga before, or not, this program is a great place to start. These fundamentals create the building blocks of a sustainable practice. Also, as I like to say - when we know the rules - we know when it's appropriate to break them. And that includes breaking the "six-week" construct. Please take as long as you need before moving forward to the next session. Life on and off the mat is a spiral; the opportunity to cycle back and deepen the experience will come. Your job is to show up and keep moving forward.

The good news is that each session is designed to help lift your mood, energize the body; and start a conversation between your mind and your body.

So let's dive into the six-week program itself.

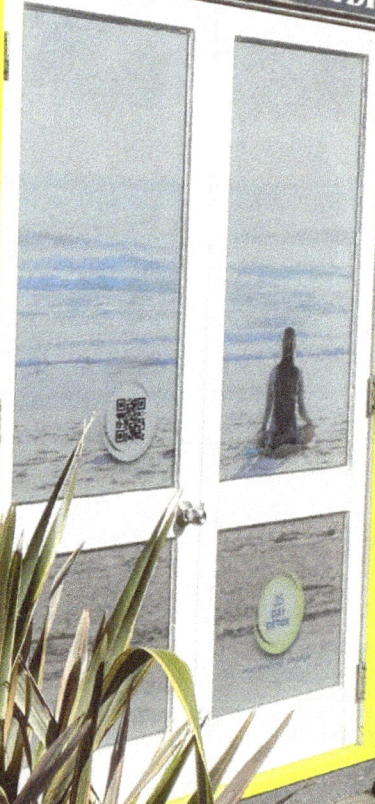

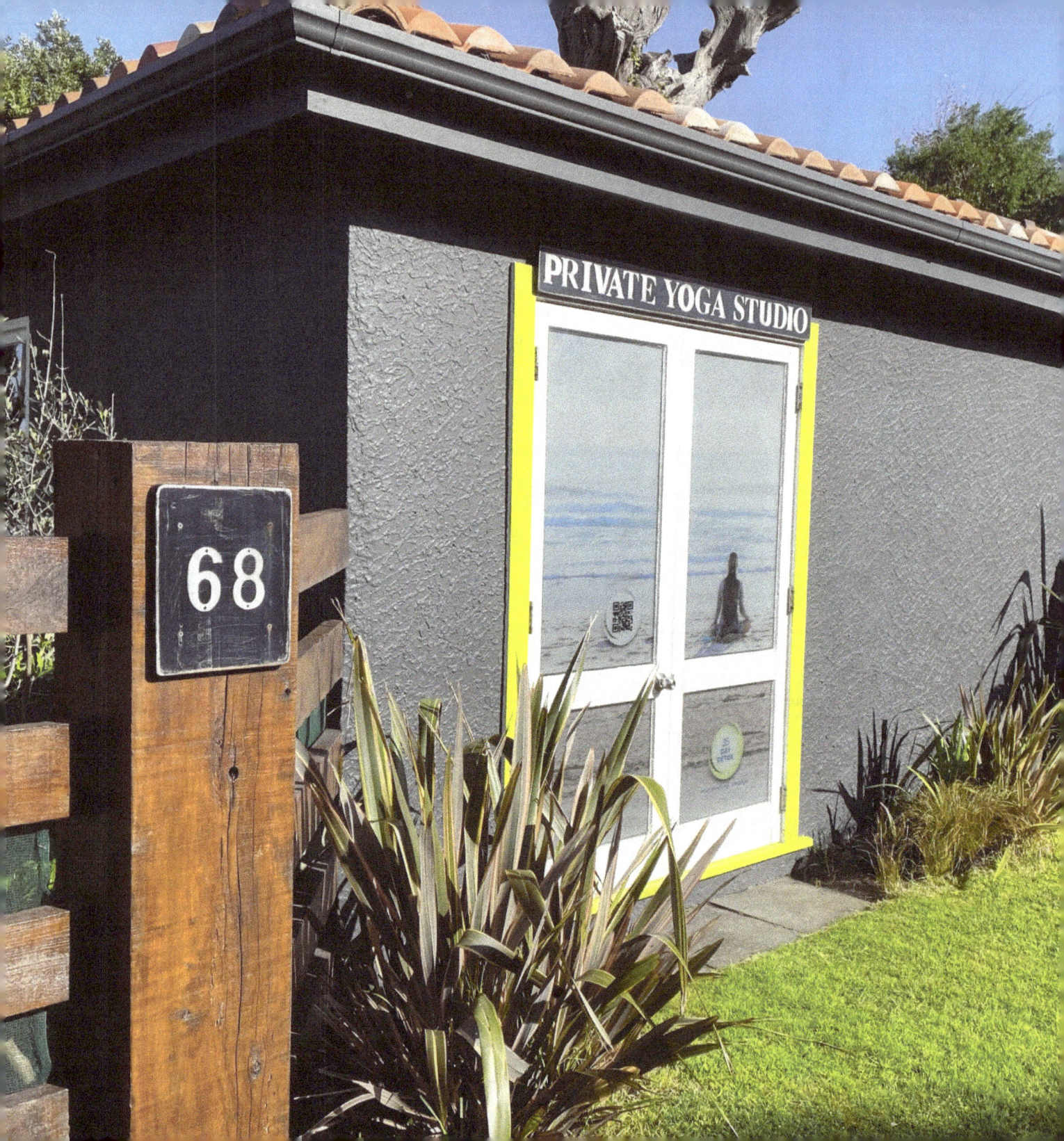

How this Program works

This book is designed to provide you with an introduction to yoga that goes deeper than attending public classes. It distills down the key elements you need to know to build the confidence to practice on your own. Knowledge is power, and once you are empowered you become your own instructor - listening to the inner guidance coming from your body. Call it intuition, or an inner knowing, this is how you create a yoga practice unique to you and your current needs.

In addition you have knowledge of what strengths and weaknesses you are bringing to the mat. I can't know that. So please be mindful of what resonates and what doesn't. Trust and back yourself to abstain from anything that doesn't feel right. Beyond this these gentle flow sessions will help uncover what you may not be consciously aware of too.

With this in mind take a moment to check in with where you are at now.

Here are my top five mobility checks as you come to the yoga studio for the first time:

1. An ability to sit upright unsupported
2. Visually check the alignment of your body for symmetry and balance (particularly shoulders and hips)
3. Standing confidently on one leg (both left and right)
4. The ability to touch your toes with knees bent
5. Gracefully get up and down to the floor (with or without hands for support)

Make a note of the things that are a struggle (or easy) and look for the yoga poses that will help you to improve. Don't forget to check both sides of the body! Ease of movement and feeling at home in your body will help you go about your daily life.

STRUCTURE OF THE SIX-WEEK PROGRAM

Each week builds on the one before. Even if you have a regular yoga practice it is worth going back to basics to reinforce what you have already learnt. It is surprising how easy it is to miss a key element of a particular pose once habit kicks in (and mindfulness is lost).

Briefly your yoga journey on this six-week program will unfold in this order.

1. The power of the Sun Salutation session to act as a warm-up and general check-in regarding the daily state of your body and mind.

2. The Stability session will centre you with the connection of the mind (giving the instructions) to the body (performing the task). Sometimes the mind is willing but the body isn't. Or potentially we are just not receiving the signals through the neural pathways.

3. Having achieved the stability to practice it is time to build the strength and flexibility in the hips and legs. This creates the foundations that allow you to expand your practice with confidence.

4. Now we can focus on building core strength. It is time to go beyond those previously limiting circumstances.

5. Next we look at the upper body and the ability to expand beyond your current situation. To truly express yourself you need the confidence that you will be supported.

6. Lastly we take the time to focus on the concept of one breath and one movement. This is also a great way to de-stress and all the changes to be integrated.

Each weekly session has a short video practice available on the website "35daydetox.com" with it's corresponding lesson focus, that you can use as the basis of a daily practice. The videos are 20 minutes but I suggest you pause and repeat sequences that resonate - and conversely skip past the ones that are inappropriate for you.

WHAT YOU WILL LEARN

42 key Yoga Poses – known as Asana in Sanskrit. The Sanskrit name is included for reference, as in some lineages of yoga they refer to poses by a different name.

Each week the focus is on seven key poses, explaining how to do them, and why they are important. These are the poses that I use time and time again when new clients come to the studio. They may not be the most "insta" worthy but they will be the most powerful starting points in rebuilding your physical being. They combine the three main benefits of strength, flexibility and balance in various combinations. Beyond that they strongly work at realigning your body, stimulating the lymphatic system, kick-starting the digestive system, unblocking energy meridians, and calming the mind.

What's missing are the back-bending poses! As a general rule I stay away from teaching them until there is the confidence, strength and stability to support that powerful part of a yoga practice. So often we sabotage our progress by over-reaching our potential. Slow and steady creates sustainable progress on and off the mat.

Every body is different. And at different times you will be different too. I can't stress this enough. We do not always arrive on the mat energised and ready to practice. These times will be the most transformative if you are willing to "JUST" show up.

WHAT'S THE DIFFERENCE BETWEEN YOGA AND A FITNESS ROUTINE?

- It's the breath! In yoga we focus on breath coordinated with movement, thus providing you with the gateway connection between the mind and body. The conversation between the body and the mind becomes two-way, allowing insight into your true state of health.
- It's also the attitude we hold to the activity. The gym mentality of "no pain no gain" gives way here to the first principle of yoga "Ahimsa - do no harm". Do no harm to others but equally importantly do no harm to yourself.
- Lastly, and most importantly, yoga is a natural detoxification process.

STUDIO COMMENTS (FROM SUZ)

A big part of me has been very resistant to creating "classes" per se. The true power of yoga is the conversation you have with your own body - not by being told what to do. Yet judging by the number of yoga studios and classes held each week around the globe I feel as if I'm the one out of step with this belief.

Reflecting on my own yoga journey I stand by my belief that it is a truth. But first we need to know how to do yoga (acquired knowledge) to empower that decision making. I had been attending classes for less than a year when I rocked up to my first Yoga Teacher Training course. In hindsight that was perfect for me as it gave me the "why" behind each of the poses and sequences. And my logical left-brain needed to "know" in order to create the buy-in to the concept of taking up a regular yoga practice.

Picking up this book is the invitation to craft your own practice. Then group classes become an adjunct; a source of inspiration and motivation on your personal health journey.

MODIFICATIONS

It is important to modify your practice to consider all circumstance that impact on you.

- Physically this includes injuries and surgeries, but also medications and illness.
- Equally importantly is the state of your emotional body. In fact I cannot stress this enough - if you are stressed or anxious then the practice needs to counter this not add to it. Check in with your heart - as it beats harder and faster you are adding to your stress levels and it is time to use a calming pose such as "extended child's pose".
- I do suggest a strength or balance pose as the antidote to an over-thinking mind. Try letting your mind drift when you are focused on holding a position, or standing on one leg! Look out for these poses in the sessions and notice the shift in your brain activity.
- Very often I will suggest a massage before beginning regular yoga. If you have knotted muscles then stretching without first releasing them is the equivalent of pulling a knot in a rubber-band. It will just make the knot tighter and almost impossible to undo. Another option is to drag out the foam roller!
- The use of body weight-bearing exercises helps with positive aging though improved bone density.

STUDIO CUES

Throughout the program you will see some cues incessantly.

- The first is to "breathe". The poses are held for too long to hold your breath! Also, we are looking to allow the body to relax and feel safe in that pose. With deep even breathing you will stimulate the Vagus Nerve and it will send the message back to the brain that everything is OK. This is a wonderful hack for all of life - not just on the mat.
- Secondly is to "engage the core". These are the muscles at the back of the body as well as the front. We do this by pulling the belly button towards the spine. In many cases you will also benefit from tucking the tailbone under to realign the spine to neutral.
- Next it is important to note that we always work with the right side of the body first. This relates to the ascending (right) and descending (left) colon of the digestive system. By starting with the right we are helping to facilitate the nature flow of waste from the body. Energetically we are working with the Yang (action) side of the body first to initiate change before the Yin (receptive) side can integrate the changes.
- Wear comfortable stretchy clothes. Practice with bare feet and remove glasses if possible. I have "a bee in my bonnet" about the tight yoga pants we all wear. These may look good but do not allow full extension of the stomach for belly breathing, and fail to allow the digestive and reproductive organs room to move.
- Be mindful of the "feet to floor", "fingertips to floor/mat", and "forehead to mat" cues; these are valuable moments of acupressure.
- Many of the poses can be approached in different ways. e.g. Mountain is a standing pose, but it can be done seated (on the floor, a chair), kneeling, as well as lying on your back (reclined).
- Find a warm quiet environment, a cold room stops the muscles and you from relaxing, and a noisy space ensures we are distracted and not present in the practice.
- There are two schools of thought on the addition of music, it provides a frequency that can enhance the state you are wishing to obtain, or it can be the distraction that stops your ability to hear the inner guidance.
- Lastly all sequences start with "hands to heart" - Anjali Mudra in Sanskrit. The palms of the hands are placed together in front of the chest, and the thumbs gently press in, connecting to the Heart Chakra. We honor the inner self who is practicing today, drawing the new energy into our physical, emotional and mental bodies with every action.

With the introductions out of the way, let's get ready to practice ...

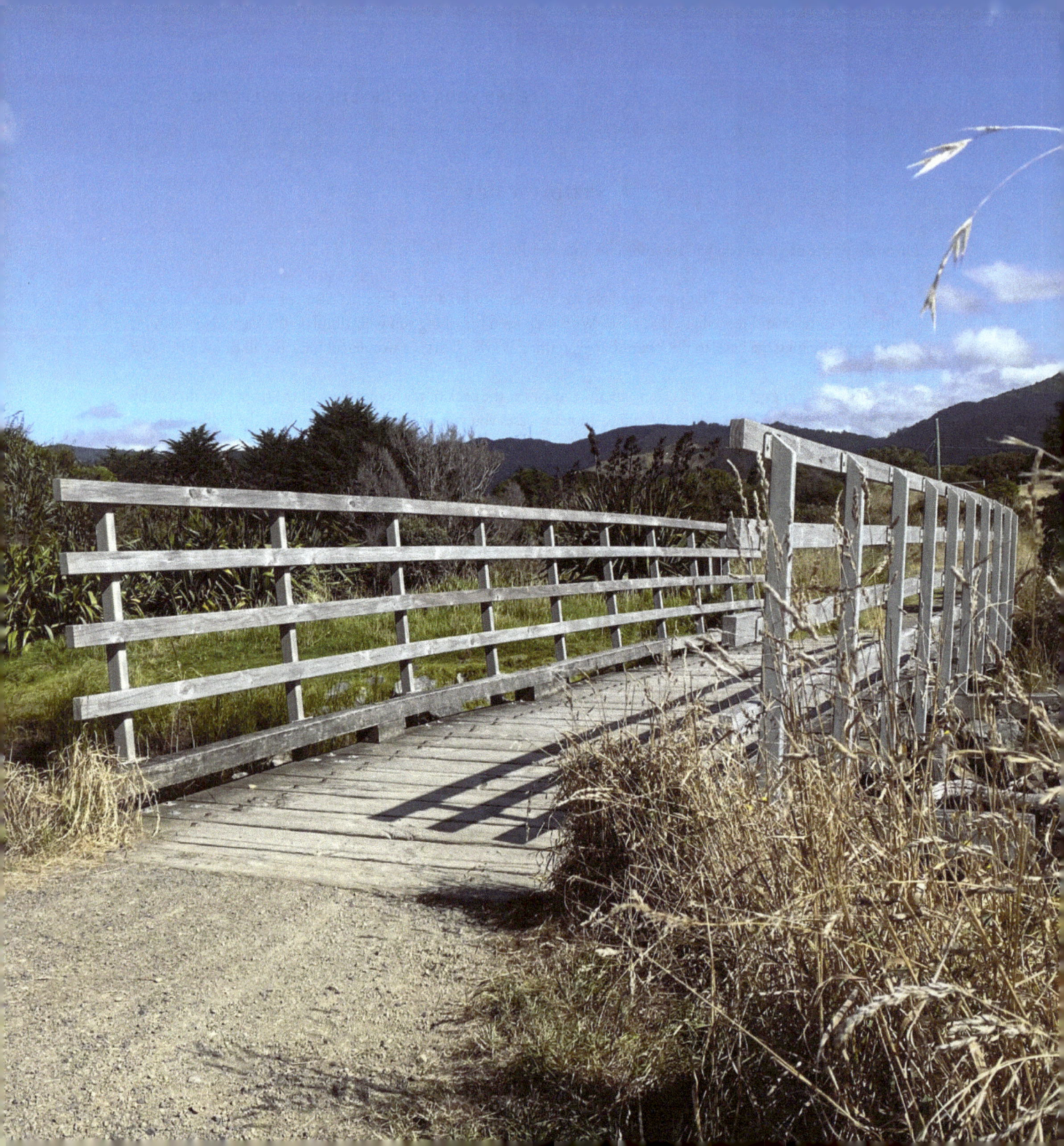

WEEK ONE - the Sun Salutation
session

The Sun Salutation (SS) sequence - Surya Namaskar in Sanskrit - is the bedrock of yoga FLOW classes. Designed to move your body from vertical to horizontal (and back), there seems to be as many versions as there are yoga teachers. What the SS sequence does is create a washing machine effect on your energy field. That gentle agitation is perfect for shaking off lethargy and starting your day energised.

The Sun rises each morning - oblivious to the dramas of the day before - and impervious to the clouds that may or may not be blocking it's light. As we turn East and practise this ancient yogic greeting of the Sun, we have an opportunity to change our experience of the day and write a new outcome.

STUDIO COMMENTS

1. The most important thing is to find a sequence that works for you at this time. As you will be doing this without a warmup it's important that is can be done without too much strain - especially if you have injuries - or are rebuilding physical fitness.

15

2. Almost everyone benefits from dropping to their knees for (modified) Plank pose on the first round of the SS. This gives the wrists and shoulders a chance to warmup before becoming fully body weight-bearing.

3. Tight hips and a weak core can make a single step forward difficult. Begin with multiple small steps, dropping the weight back, and coming onto the fingertips until you have control of the forward momentum. Alternatively you can walk your hands to your feet until you have the core strength to make this transition comfortably.

4. An important part of the yoga practice is the moment of stillness at the end of the practice (even after 10 minutes). Jumping up and off the mat doesn't allow time for integration and can leave you feeling unbalanced, skittish or exhausted for the rest of the day.

THE SEQUENCE EXPLAINED

Stand steady, inhale and reach for the sky in **Mountain (pose)**, exhale reach down to the earth in **Forward Fold**, inhale and look forward to a **Half Lift**, exhale step back leading with the right leg to **Plank**, drop to your knees and lower all the way to the mat, inhale and lift the chin and chest to **Cobra**, exhale to come back to the floor, push up to the knees and lift the hips to **Downdog**, inhale and step forward leading with the right leg to **Half Lift**, exhale **Forward Fold**, inhale reach tall again to **Mountain**, exhale hands to heart or to the sides of the body. Repeat leading with the left leg. This is one round, do between 3–5 rounds to warmup fully.

PRACTICE SEQUENCE

To become familiar with the Sun Salutation sequence it helps to break it down and repeat sections. It is also a great way to get the body moving - especially as you are just beginning this journey. e.g. Group the standing poses together and repeat them 3-5 times. Then move down to the mat and do the floor-based poses 3-5 times separately. Another option is to add one or two poses to the SS sequence to make it a complete yoga session. e.g. consider adding a **High Lunge** after **Downdog** to work on stability and presence.

BONUS MATERIAL

The reality is that often we skip our simple yoga routine in the morning. We are distracted, in a rush, the reasons are endless, and valid! What I generally say in response to this is - it is very unlikely that you will have skipped cleaning your teeth. So, enter the body floss, a gentle **Twisting Warmup** that can be done every day!

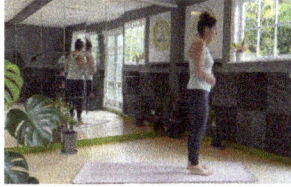

Twisting Warmup

CONSIDER THIS A FLOSSING OF THE WHOLE BODY. JUST
AS YOU FLOSS YOUR TEETH EACH MORNING TO REMOVE
THE BUILDUP OF PLAQUE.

STUDIO CUES

- Make sure you haven't eaten for at least an hour
- Stand feet hip width apart with a slight bend in the knees
- Soften the eye gaze so that you are not externally focused
- Bring hands to belly and at your own pace start to gently twist side-to-side
- Release hands to fully twist including the shoulder and neck in the movement
- To stop, slow down before coming into stillness

BENEFITS

- Relieves physical tension in neck, upper back, hips and legs
- Improves blood flow and lymphatic circulation
- Creates a moving meditation, focus inwards to calm the mind and centre the body

MODIFICATIONS

- Feeling dizzy, don't stop immediately, slow and then come into stillness

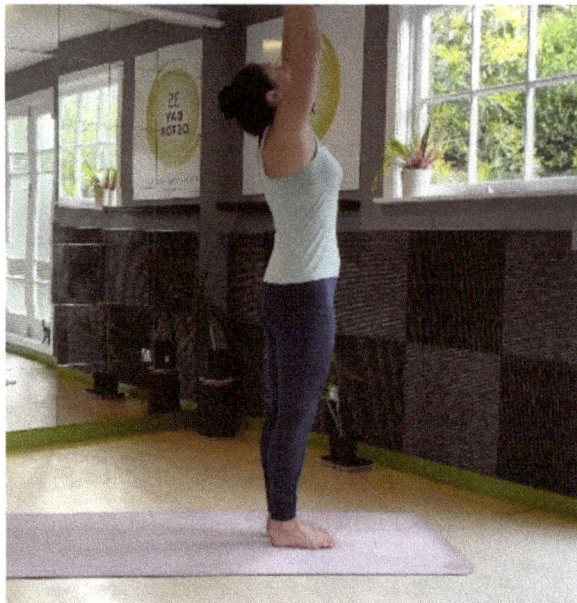

Mountain Pose
(Tadasana)

STANDING TALL WITH THE SOVEREIGNTY OF THE
MOUNTAIN, YET NOTICE SMALL MOVEMENTS NECESSARY
TO ADJUST TO EVER-MOVING SURROUNDING ENERGIES.

STUDIO CUES

- Stand feet hip width apart or "big toes together and heels apart", hands together at the heart, pull the kneecaps up
- Tuck the tailbone under by tilting the pelvis forward and engage the core by pulling belly button to spine
- Raise the arms overhead keeping the arms straight, elbows close to the ears and shoulders are down
- Hands are parallel directly above the shoulders or palms together

BENEFITS

- Become present, develop an awareness of your physical being
- Improve posture
- Achieve better overall balance
- Relieve sciatic pain
- Improve breathing by deepening the lung's capacity
- Invigorate the body and mind, shaking off lethargy

MODIFICATIONS

- If balance is an issue focus your eyes on a non-moving point straight ahead
- Use the peripheral vision to watch as you raise the arms overhead
- Make it more challenging by rising onto the toes as the arms go overhead
- This overhead stretch can also be done seated on a chair, kneeling, or lying on your back (on the floor or bed)
- If shoulder mobility is an issue bring the arms forward and work with your current range.

PARTNER WITH:
STANDING SIDE STRETCHES,
FORWARD FOLD AND HALF LIFT POSES

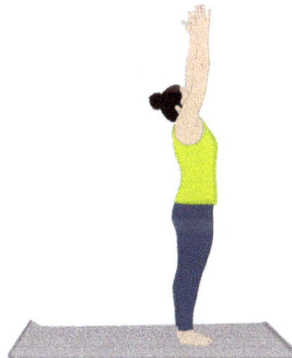

Mountain Pose

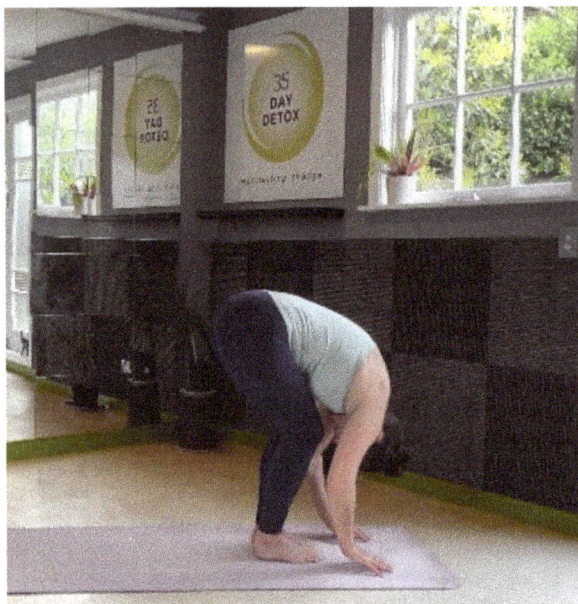

Forward Fold Pose
(Uttanasana)

BOW TO GREET EARTH AND RELEASE NEED FOR CONTROL.
AS HEAD DROPS BELOW HEART TRUST THAT YOUR BODY
INSTINCTIVELY KNOWS WHAT IS RIGHT.

STUDIO CUES
- Begin standing with feet hip width apart and hands on hips
- Fold from the hips leading with the chin and chest to maintain a flat back
- Engage the core as you fold, bend knees to reduce the impact of the hamstring stretch
- Drop the head and look towards the knees, deepen the stretch by leaning slightly forward

BENEFITS

- Relieve pressure on the lower back
- Release tension in the neck
- Calms the mind
- Stimulates digestion
- Creates an improved sense of wellbeing

MODIFICATIONS

- If you suffer from low blood pressure, dizziness, or a lack of balance, bend the knees more and keep the head above the shoulders with the eye gaze to the mat
- Create a longer deep hold by placing hands to elbows and using the weight of the upper body to stretch further
- Practice this forward fold seated on a chair

PARTNER WITH:
MOUNTAIN, HALF LIFT, DOWNDOG
AND PYRAMID POSES

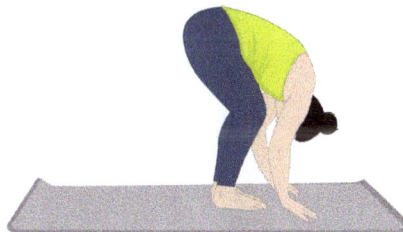

Forward Fold Pose

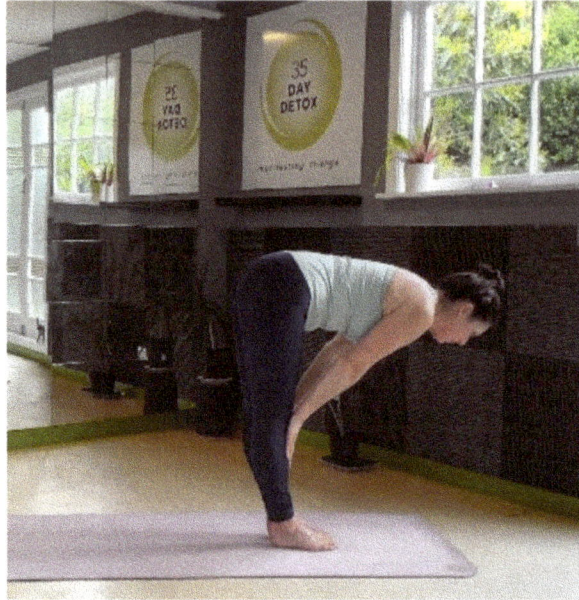

Half Lift Pose
(Ardha Uttanasana)

HALFWAY BETWEEN THE SKY AND EARTH IS OUR PHYSICAL PRESENCE. LEAD WITH YOUR HEART AND BE CONFIDENT IN YOUR BODY TO SUPPORT YOUR LIFE.

STUDIO CUES

- Stand legs hip width apart and hands on hips, fold from the hips with straight legs
- Press hands to legs and lengthen through the spine, pull shoulders down away from ears
- Relax the neck and look directly down to the mat, lean slightly into the toes with heels on the ground

BENEFITS

- Stretches hamstrings and hip muscles
- Improves posture and spinal alignment
- Develops balance and spatial awareness
- Can alleviate menopause symptoms

MODIFICATIONS

- Start with hands on or below the knees until you can comfortably place fingertips to floor
- At night this pose can be flipped to become "legs up the wall", a restorative and regenerative experience of spinal realignment

PARTNER WITH:
MOUNTAIN, FORWARD FOLD AND PYRAMID POSES

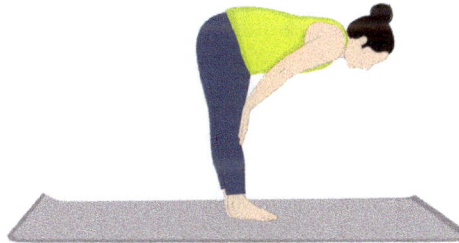

Half Lift Pose

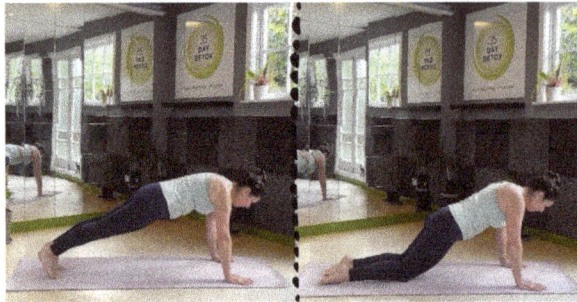

Plank Pose
(Phalakasana)

PRESS YOUR HANDS INTO THE EARTH TO RECEIVE
STRENGTH TO CARRY YOURSELF FROM ONE SITUATION
TO ANOTHER.

STUDIO CUES

- Start kneeling with hands below shoulders and knees below hips (this is **Tabletop** pose)
- Straighten the right leg and place toes on floor, repeat with the left leg
- Body (including head) is now in one long line, push through heels and pull kneecaps up
- Keep arms strong and shoulders back, engage core muscles by pulling belly button to spine
- Drop to the knees without shifting the shoulder position for modified plank

BENEFITS

- Strengthens shoulders, arms and wrists
- Tones core muscles
- Builds confidence
- Tames the mind

MODIFICATIONS

- Almost everyone benefits from dropping to the knees in modified plank until warmed up
- Alternatively practice with pushing a single leg back and engaging the core. Progress to hover the kneeling leg slightly off the floor
- Take the practice away from the mat and into daily life, use a solid structure (such as a bench) to build strength without loading the wrists

PARTNER WITH:
DOWNDOG, COBRA, EXTENDED CHILD'S POSE,
THREAD THE NEEDLE AND WRIST RELEASES

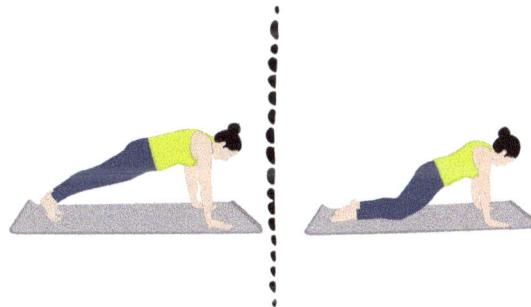

Plank and Modified Plank Poses

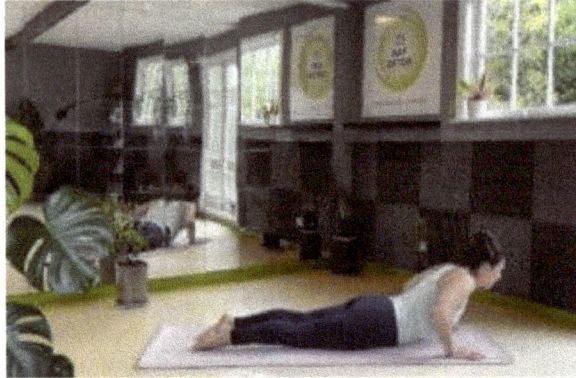

Cobra Pose
(Bhujangasana)

DROP DOWN TO RELEASE TENSION. LIFT YOUR HEART TO
GREET THE SUN AND RECEIVE IT'S ENERGY FOR THE DAY.

STUDIO TIPS

- Lie on your stomach with legs hip width apart, point through the toes and pull heels inwards
- Elbows are bent and hands and wrists are directly under shoulders
- Keep the elbows tucked in to the side body, press through the hands to lift chin and chest from the mat
- Engage the back muscles to hold you without clenching the gluteal muscles (buttocks)

BENEFITS

- Strengthen the lower back muscles
- Counteracts too much sitting
- Energise the mind
- Stimulates the digestive and reproductive organs
- Alleviate menstrual discomfort
- Balance hormones

MODIFICATIONS

- Find your natural height of the chest lift by removing the hands from the mat and hold that position
- Protect your lower back by limiting the lift of the upper body until you have the strength in the back muscles
- Add breath and movement by exhaling to twist and look over your shoulder, inhale back to centre, then exhale to the other side, inhale to centre, exhale back to the mat

PARTNER WITH:
EXTENDED CHILD'S POSE, CAT COW AND PUPPY POSE

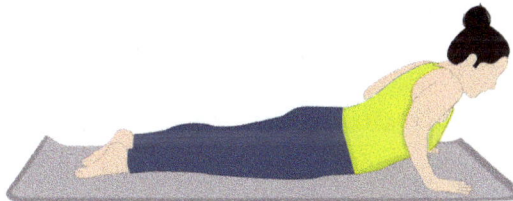

Cobra Pose

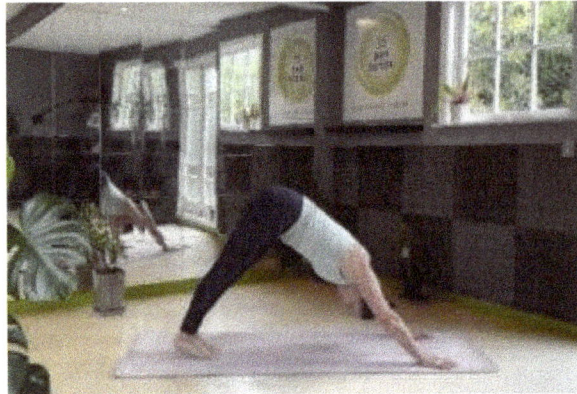

Downdog Pose
(Adho Mukha Svanasana)

AS YOUR HEAD DROPS BELOW THE HEART BE PREPARED TO
SEE LIFE FROM A NEW PERSPECTIVE.

STUDIO CUES

- From **Tabletop** pose move the hands forward a hand length to create a stable base
- Stretch fingers wide with middle finger pointed forward to activate pressure points in the fingers and palms
- Hands are shoulder width apart and feet hip width apart,
- Push through hands to stretch through the spine as you lift the hips high
- Drop heels towards the floor and pull the kneecaps up to stretch the back of the legs
- Look to the knees

BENEFITS

- Full body stretch
- Relieves stress and tension
- Strengthens shoulders
- Stretches calf muscles
- Improves blood circulation

MODIFICATIONS

- If dizziness or vertigo is an issue keep the eye gaze to the mat
- Deepen the stretch by gently pushing one heel after the other to the mat in a walking motion
- Challenge yourself to place one foot on the other heel for 3-5 breaths

PARTNER WITH:
EXTENDED CHILD'S POSE, PLANK, WILD THING
AND TWISTED LUNGE POSES

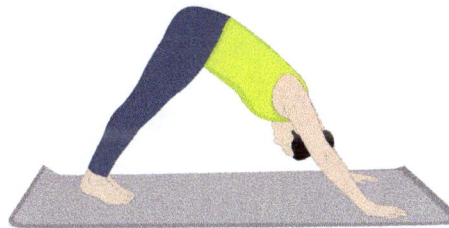

Downdog Pose

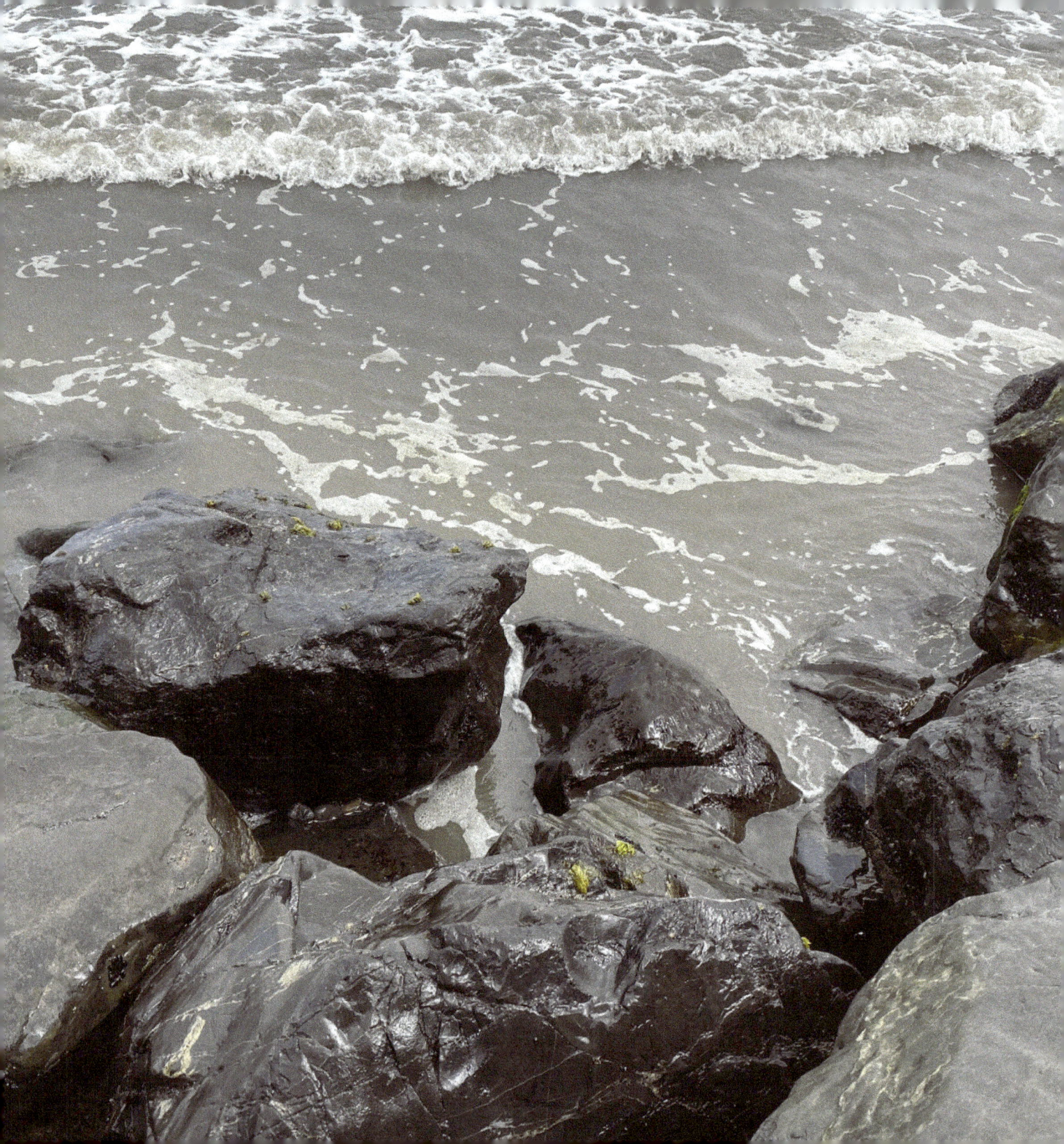

WEEK TWO - finding Stability and Balance

Before anything in yoga it is important to connect to your body. Often we are blissfully unaware of what is happening under the skin. That is until something goes wrong and then all attention is on that issue. What I have found in the studio is that whatever symptom is manifest has underlying causes. And very often those causes come back to a misalignment on the body, most often stemming from a childhood injury or trauma.

Use the analog of a car - most of us get in and start the engine - we expect the car to take us where we want to go. Probably the user manual is that last thing we think to consult. So let's get onto the mat and begin the dialog between mind and body - accessing the innate knowledge of how your body really functions.

STUDIO COMMENTS

1. With single leg balancing take the practice off the mat. Find opportunities within your daily activities to stand on one leg. My favourites include - waiting for the kettle to boil, cleaning your teeth, standing in a queue (with the proviso that you are wearing flat shoes).

2. A steady eye gaze will help to still the mind. Simply put, there are less images for the brain to process. Gently place the big toe on the floor, until you develop the balance (this is more effective than falling out of the pose multiple times).

3. Similarly place a fingertip (or two) on a fixed object until you build the strength and confidence to stand unsupported.

4. Consider the three planes of the body - vertical, horizontal, and diagonal. There is a pivot point (centre of gravity) available to you in each. As you find that "centre" internally you will become stable externally too.

PRACTICE SEQUENCE

You are focusing on creating stability by activating the core muscles (including hips). Equally importantly is the mindfulness that goes with a gentle practice connecting breath and movement. This session you will practice single leg balance as well as kneeling balance poses. It is a combination of strength and flexibility to create confidence in your sense of balance and stability.

Use the SS sequence to warmup first. Return to the front of the mat with hands to heart. Take a few calming breaths, allowing the heart-rate to drop and the breathing to become slow and even once more. Choose either (or both) standing poses - **Tree** and/or **Standing Side Stretches**. Come down to the mat for the kneeling poses - **Cat Cow, Low Lunge**, and **Kneeling Superman**. Finish with **Extended Child's** pose. Take time at the end of the session (or before bed in the evening) to spend a few minutes lying in **Relaxation Meditation**.

BONUS MATERIAL

To assist in making that connection between Mind and Body I offer an easy 10 minute guided relaxation meditation that you can do any time of the day. It combines belly breathing with body awareness. It's a very simple way to bring you out of your mind-space and connect to the innate knowledge of the body.

As we slow down our physical activities, thoughts, and breath we hear that intuitive voice in a stronger way. In fact the main reason yogis do the daily physical practice (asana) is so that they can sit in comfort for meditation, tapping into that inner wisdom.

Relaxation Meditation

Here's an easy 10 minute guided relaxation that you can do any time of the day. It combines belly breathing with body awareness. It's a very simple way to bring you out of your mind-space and connect to the innate knowledge of the body.

STUDIO CUES

- Find a warm comfortable position where you won't be interrupted
- Ensure your clothes are not tight around the abdomen
- Lie on your back with legs hip width apart
- Let the feet relax and fall slightly out
- Bring arms beside the hips with palms facing up
- Tuck the chin in and have head to floor (or a low cushion)

TRANSCRIPT

Connect body and mind through the awareness of the breath. Close your eyes and take a deep breath in through the nose, and a clearing breath out through the mouth (repeat twice more). Remain with eyes closed and body in stillness. Begin to bring your awareness to different parts of your body.

Start at the feet, wiggle the toes, feel the energies in the toes. Check in at the ankles, notice how they feel. Now the calf muscles, the right and then the left. Check in with the knees, and then the thighs. See if one leg feels higher than the other. Do they feel like they are in balance, or skewed to one side. Make any slight physical adjustments now.

Come into the hip area. Feel a connection to the earth through the buttocks to the floor. Make sure you are evenly connected. Relax into the hip and pelvic area. Move up to the stomach area. Is the stomach moving with the breath. Notice if the diaphragm is working.

Relax the upper back, chest and shoulders. Notice the shoulders, is one hitched up tighter than the other. Make any adjustments.

Come to the neck and throat area - travel up the back of the head, over the top to the crown of the head and forehead. Notice the tension residing there. Blink the eyes a few times to release tension. How does the jaw feel? Is the mouth closed and breathing without effort.

Return to the shoulders and arms, feel any tension draining away and leaving the body from the fingertips.

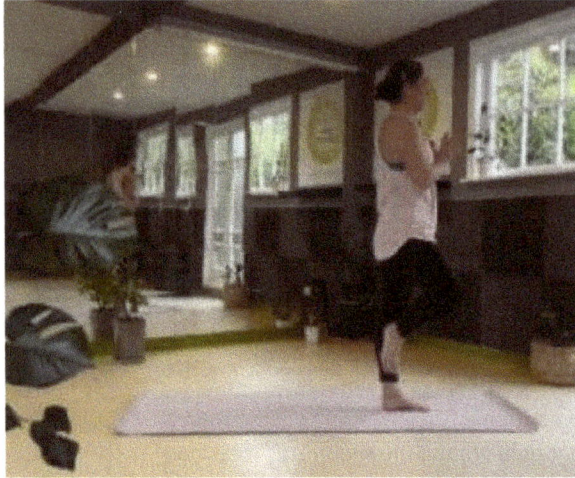

Tree Pose
(Vrksasana)

FIND STABILITY IN THE LOWER BODY TO ALLOW FULL
EXPRESSION OF WHO YOU ARE TO MANIFEST THROUGH
CREATIVE EXPRESSION.

STUDIO CUES

- Stand on a stable surface and shift the weight to the left foot
- Ensure the standing leg (ankle, knee), hip and shoulder are in one line
- Engage the core to lift the right leg, bend the knee and turn it out to the side, place the foot on the left leg
- Find a focal point that is not moving and fix your eyes on that point
- Bring hands to heart, still the mind and focus on the breath

BENEFITS

- Grounding, i.e. feeling connected to your physical life
- Calming for the mind
- Improves balance and posture

MODIFICATIONS

- Use a solid structure (wall or bench) for support
- Place the big toe on the floor until you can stand without falling out of the pose
- Aim for 5-10 breaths on each side
- Don't hesitate to return to the weaker side and repeat in order to bring your body into balance

PARTNER WITH:
MOUNTAIN, TRIANGLE, STANDING SIDE STRETCHES
AND FORWARD FOLD POSES

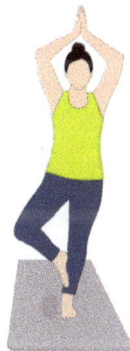

Tree Pose

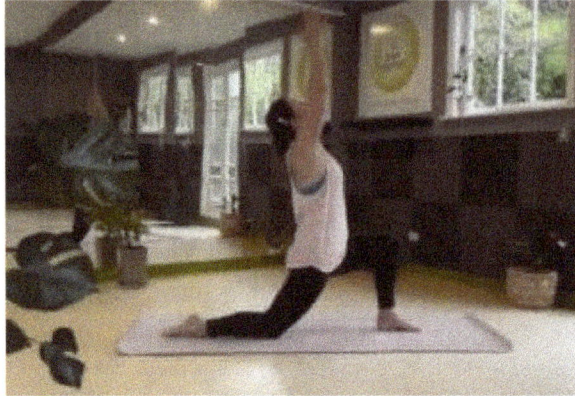

Low Lunge Pose
(Anjaneyasana)

GROUND THE FEET TO THE EARTH AND REACH FOR THE SKY. INNER GROWTH IS THE UNSEEN ROOT STRUCTURE THAT ULTIMATELY SUSTAINS US.

STUDIO CUES

- From standing (feet hip width apart), step the left leg back
- Drop the left knee to floor and point toes and flatten foot to floor
- Ensure the front knee is directly over ankle (use the hand to bring the foot further forward if necessary)
- Engage the core muscles, bring shoulders directly over the hips, raise the arms overhead
- Challenge your stability by looking up to the thumbs

BENEFITS

- Stretches the hip flexor muscles
- Release tension in the hips after sitting for long periods
- Relieves sciatic pain
- Stimulates the thyroid
- Develops inner balance and focus

MODIFICATIONS

- Remain with hands to the front thigh until you are confident with the balance
- Transition with hands to heart to correct the alignment of the torso, thereby protecting the lower back
- Challenge yourself to move into **High Lunge** by lifting the back knee off the floor

PARTNER WITH:
DOWNDOG, HALF SPLIT, TWISTED LUNGE
AND PYRAMID POSES

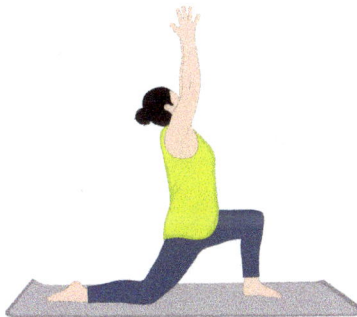

Low Lunge Pose

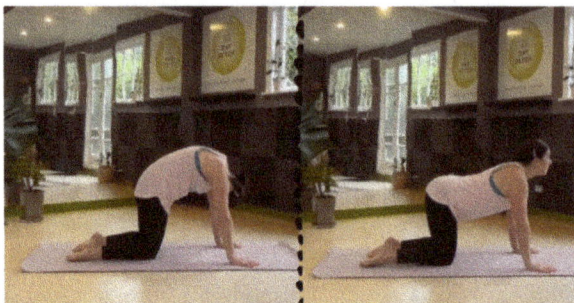

Cat Cow Pose
(Chakravakasana)

YOUR SPINE IS THE SUPER HIGHWAY OF YOUR ENERGY
SYSTEM. ALL MESSAGES ARE SENT AND RECEIVED
WITHOUT JUDGMENT.

STUDIO CUES

- Start in **Tabletop** pose, keep toes pointed and tops of the feet evenly to floor
- Exhale and move to **Cat** pose, and inhale move to **Cow** pose
- In **Cat** arch the back (lower, mid and upper) up and drop the chin to chest
- In **Cow** drop the stomach down and lift the head to feel the stretch through the front of the body
- Feel the lengthening (and movement) of the spine from neck to tailbone

BENEFITS

- Creates movement along the spine
- Improves balance
- Provides a gentle massage for the digestive and reproductive organs
- Improves hormonal system's function
- Moderates breathing to step away from a stress response

MODIFICATIONS

- Notice the connection with the breath and the movement. In a stress response you will breath in the opposite way. Stop, reset in the neutral position of T**abletop**, then begin again - this time with the exhale to **Cat** pose first
- Take the time to explore the movement in each part of the back - tailbone, lower back, mid back, upper back and neck
- The seated version on a chair (or floor) is achieved by holding the hands lightly on the knees for support

PARTNER WITH:
KNEELING SUPERMAN, PUPPY AND THREAD THE NEEDLE POSES

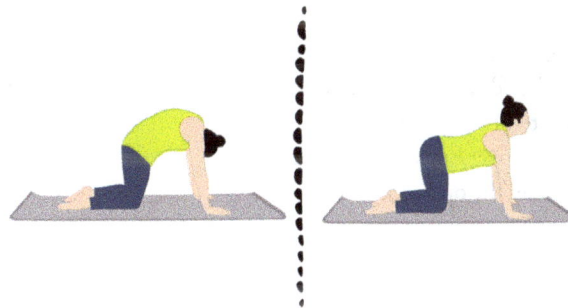

Cat Cow Pose

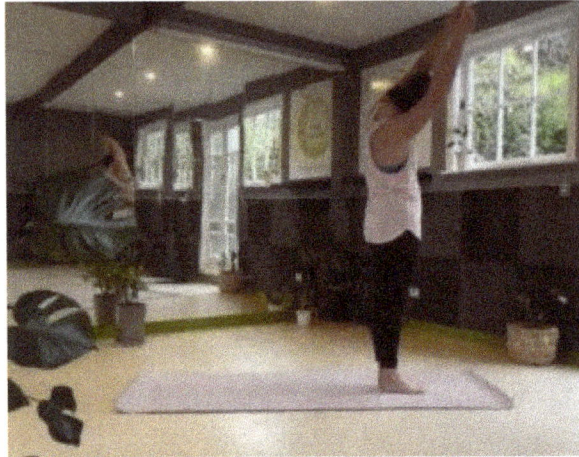

Standing Side Stretches
(Parsva Tadasana)

STRETCH OUT TO RELEASE LIMITS PREVIOUSLY PLACED ON YOU BY OTHERS AND EXPAND YOUR PRESENCE INTO NEW PLACES.

STUDIO CUES

- Begin in **Mountain** pose, raise arms overhead with fingers interlaced, thumbs crossed and index fingers together
- Exhale as you drop to the right side first, push opposite hip out to create a stretch from ankle to wrist
- Use the core (and an inhale) to bring you back to centre
- Ensure the hips don't twist or upper body fall forward
- Eye gaze straight ahead or under the opposite armpit

BENEFITS

- Improved reach (think the top shelf at the supermarket)
- Stimulate the lymphatic system
- Energise the mind

MODIFICATIONS

- Use this pose to create a breath and movement sequence. Exhale as you drop to the side and inhale back to centre.
- This side stretch can be done seated (floor or chair), as well as lying on the floor (or bed)

PARTNER WITH:
LOW LUNGE, PYRAMID AND TRIANGLE POSES

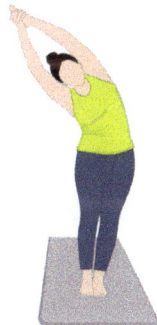

Standing Side Stretch

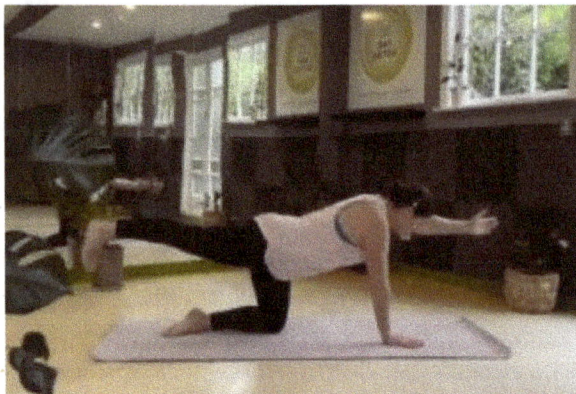

Kneeling Superman Pose / Balancing Table Pose
(Dandayamana Bharmanasana)

WE ARE CAPABLE OF MORE THAN WE GIVE OURSELVES
CREDIT FOR. HOLD STEADY AND ALLOW THE ENERGY TO
BUILD MOMENTUM.

STUDIO CUES

- Start in **Tabletop**, keep the eye gaze to the floor and neck neutral
- Lift the right leg to hip height and left arm to shoulder height, flex the foot to stabilise the leg
- Turn hand so thumb is on top and palm faces the mid-line - this rolls the shoulder open and expands the chest
- Feel as though you are being pulled simultaneously by the foot and hand to expand lengthways

BENEFITS

- Improves balance
- Develops core strength
- Strengthens wrists, arms and shoulders

MODIFICATIONS

- Bring knees and hands a little closer to the mid-line for extra stability
- Challenge yourself by bringing the hand and foot out to a 45 degree angle
- Keep both leg and arm in line with the body

PARTNER WITH:
THREAD THE NEEDLE, EXTENDED CHILD'S POSE WITH SIDE STRETCHES
AND WRIST RELEASES

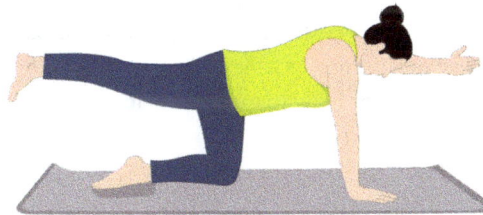

Kneeling Superman Pose

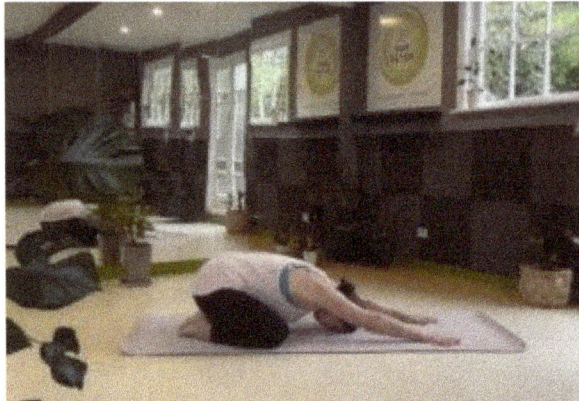

Extended Child's Pose
(Utthita Balasana)

SURRENDER ALL THOUGHTS AND TENSIONS TO MOTHER EARTH. ALLOW TIME FREEDOM TO REIGN SUPREME.

STUDIO CUES

- Kneel with big toes together and knees as wide as comfortable
- Sink buttocks back to sit on the heels (use a cushion behind the knees for extra support)
- Slide hands forward to floor stretching the fingers wide
- Drop the forehead to the floor and sink the body towards the mat

BENEFITS

- Provides respite and recovery during the yoga practice
- Improves sleep by relaxing the body and mind
- Stimulates the digestive system
- Acts as an emotional release
- Relief for lower back tension

MODIFICATIONS

- Alternatively stack the hands to provide support for the neck
- If bending the knee is an issue then keep the hips high with the foot out to the side
- Contain the energy within by bringing the thumbs and index fingers gently together

PARTNER WITH:
ALL POSES

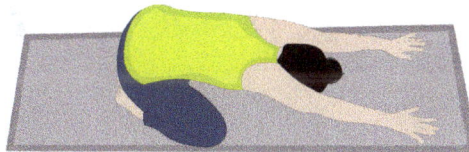

Extended Child's Pose

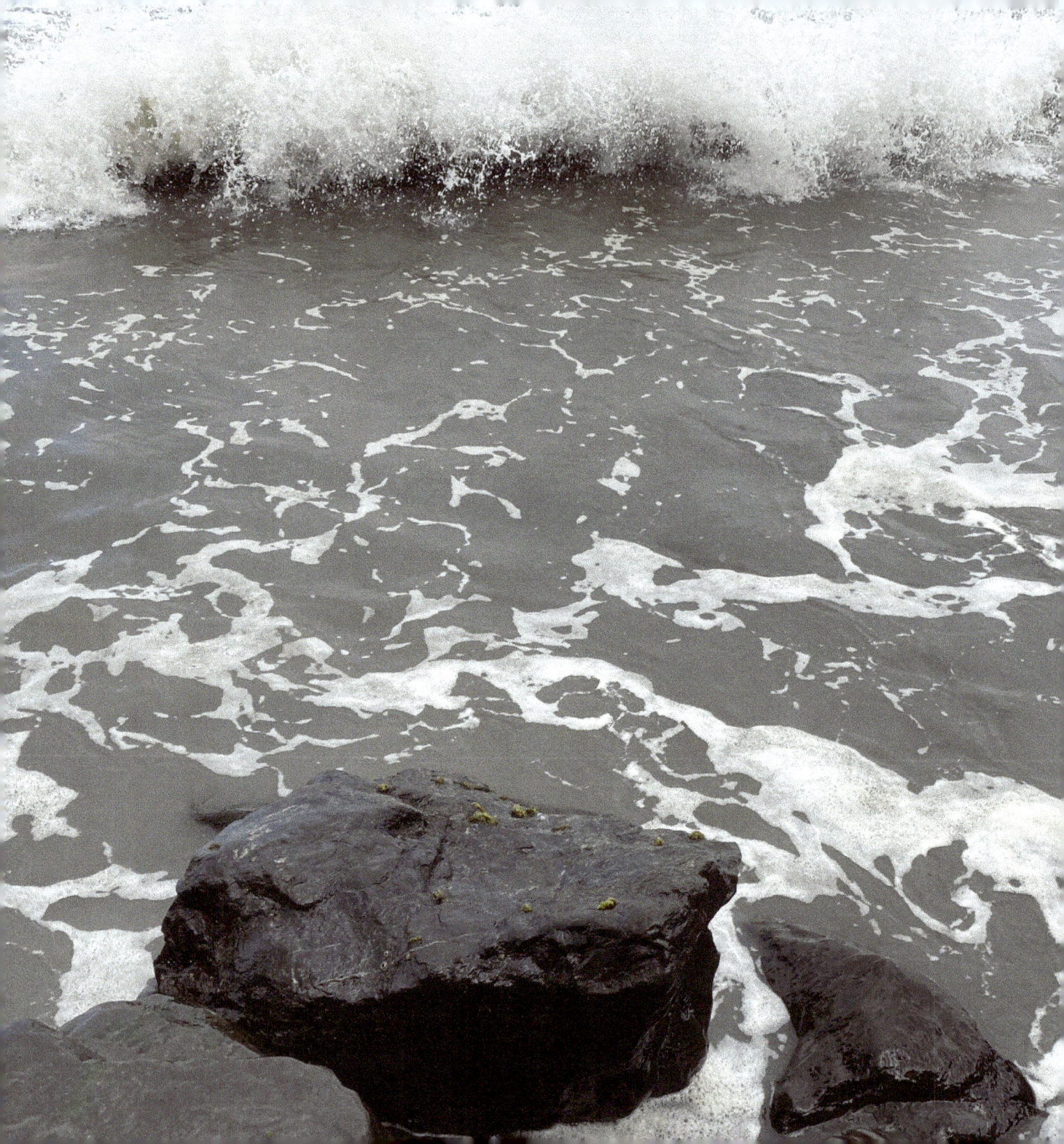

WEEK THREE - building Strong Foundations

Like the building that will be only as good as the foundations - so too our bodies. Having developed a sense of stability with the previous week's session we can move onto creating stronger foundations. Those foundations - like the roots of a tree - are the joints (feet, ankles, knees, hips) and leg muscles.

A STABLE BASE IS REQUIRED TO SUPPORT ANY GROWTH. WITHIN OUR ENERGITIC BODY THAT IS THE REALM OF THE FIRST CHAKRA. THE RIGHT TO A WARM SAFE ENVIRONMENT WITH SUFFICIENT FOOD. INSECURITY LEADS TO INSTABILITY AND CREATES A STRESS RESPONSE. STRUCTURE AND DISCIPLINE HELP BUILD STRONG FOUNDATIONS.

STUDIO COMMENTS

1. In all the poses you will simultaneously do both strengthening and flexibility. These are the opposing forces that keep you in balance. e.g. As you stretch the hamstrings you will strengthen the quad muscles, as you stretch the lower back muscles you will activate the stomach muscles. Be mindful of both parts of the equation in all the poses.

2. This week's focus is on your hips and legs. The route to improvement is not a straight line, so be prepared to work the split-stance (with two feet on the mat) to create improvement that will feed back to the single leg poses.

3. Developing mobility in the lower joints (ankles and knees) will take the pressure of the larger hip joints.

4. It is a great option to group the dynamic standing poses in the morning to energise you for the day.

5. This leaves the kneeling and seated poses in the evening to release the tensions of the day. They help calm the mind and prepare you for a restful night's sleep.

LEG PAIN

Generalised leg pain often stems from tightness in the muscles, perhaps it's been a long time since the legs were truly relaxed. So much so that we are only aware of the tension when we begin to stretch them. Preferable not to stretch then? No, time to do something more. The YIN yoga style of "legs up the wall" is ideal to release that tension, realign the spine, and reduce puffiness around the joints.

PRACTICE SEQUENCE

In this week's gentle flow yoga session you will focus on your hips and legs.

It is a good time to introduce the "mandala" flow. This style of sequence adds one or two more poses to the sequence each time. Building on what went before! And is a lovely way to remember longer sequences. As an added bonus, you will likely finding yourself beginning to extend the length of time on mat.

Start with the SS sequence warmup, 1-3 rounds to ensure you have connected breath and movement. Next practice **Tree** pose to centre you into the present moment. Move onto the hip/leg sequence - from the front of the mat do 3 sets of **Standing Side Stretches**. Step back to **Low Lunge** and then lift the back knee to **Twisted Lunge**. Come back to the front of the mat and repeat for the left side. Next round drop the back knee to the floor to add **Half Split** and **High Lunge** before stepping forward to the front of the mat. On the final round add a step halfway up the mat for **Pyramid,** followed by the **Half Lift**. Next come down to a seated position on the mat for **Butterfly, Head Beyond Knee** and **Half Spinal Twist**. Lastly spend time lying on your back for **Relaxation Meditation**.

By creating a strong foundation you can approach life with greater ease and confidence.

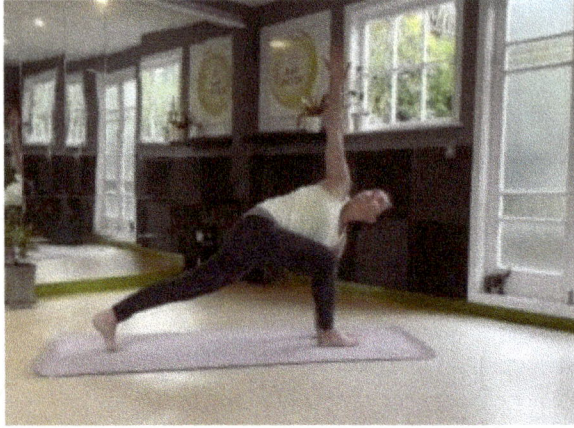

Twisted Lunge Pose
(Parivrtta Anjenayasana)

CONSIDER NEW WAYS TO SEE THE WORLD AS YOU TWIST
AND CONFRONT AN OLD VIEWPOINT.

STUDIO CUES

- From standing, bend the knees, place hands on the floor and step the left leg back
- Stay on the toes of the back foot, push the heel back and pull the kneecap up to straighten the back leg
- Keep the front knee bent and ensure it is directly over the ankle
- Press left hand to the floor under shoulder and beside the right foot, stack shoulder over shoulder in one line
- Palm is open, facing away from the body, fingers stretched wide
- Engage the core and pull right knee gently towards the body
- Look up to the right thumb

BENEFITS

- Builds strength in the legs
- Stretches the hip flexor muscles
- Stimulates digestive system
- Develops balance and confidence

MODIFICATIONS

- Stay with the knee to the ground (in **Low Lunge**) until you develop balance and leg strength
- If you have shoulder injuries try placing the top arm gently behind the back rather than reaching high

**PARTNER WITH:
HIGH LUNGE, EAGLE, PYRAMID
AND DOWNDOG POSES**

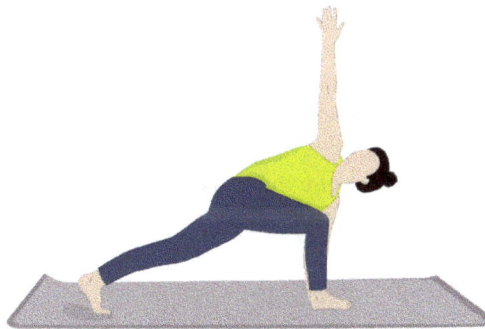

Twisted Lunge Pose

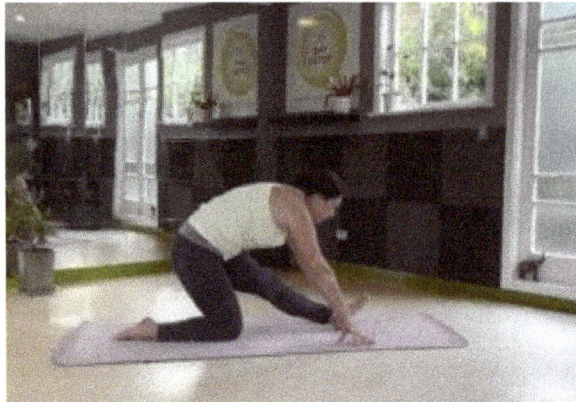

Half Split Pose
(Ardha Hanumanasana)

PULL BACK TO LEAP FORWARD. OUT OF SIGHT - OUT OF MIND - ONLY WORKS TO HOLD THE STATUS QUO.

STUDIO CUES

- From **Low Lunge** pose, place hands beside the right front foot on floor for support
- Hips drop back past the left knee but stay raised
- As you fold forward over the leg lead with the chin and chest to maintain a flat back
- Eye gaze is forward past the foot
- Flex the front foot to stretch the calf, then point through the toes to stretch the muscles around the shin

BENEFITS

- Classic hamstring stretch!
- Improves range of motion of the hips, creating a sense of lightness and agility
- Releases tension in the hips and legs
- Provides a feeling of being grounded and a sense of security

MODIFICATIONS

- Use yoga blocks or books if you can't place fingertips on the floor yet
- Make a stretch dynamic by inhaling into **Low Lunge** and exhaling to **Half Split**
- Stretch the hamstrings whilst seated on a chair, straighten the right leg and flex the foot

PARTNER WITH:
DOWNDOG, KNEELING HIP RELEASES, LOW LUNGE
AND PYRAMID POSES

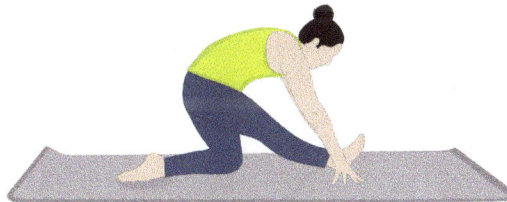

Half Split Pose

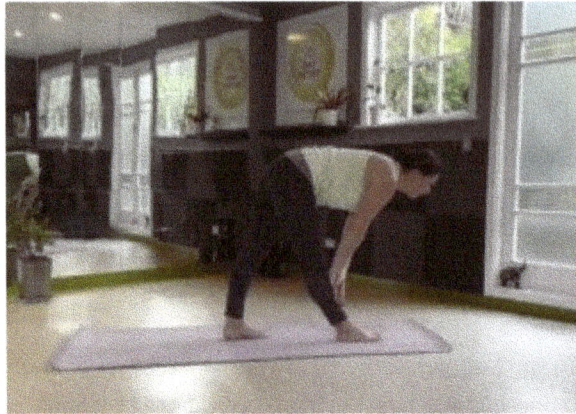

Pyramid Pose
(Parsvottanasana)

FIND EQUILIBRIUM IN BOTH STRENGTH AND FLEXIBILITY TO HOLD THE SPACE BETWEEN TWO OPPOSING POINTS OF VIEW.

STUDIO CUES

- Begin standing with feet hip width apart, take a small step back with the left foot to set up the right-side pose
- Ensure the knees don't bend, keep engaging the leg muscles by pulling the kneecaps up
- Use the hands on the hips to check that both hips are level and not twisting
- Fold from the hips, leading with the chin and chest to keep the back flat
- When you have reached the end of your range-of-motion place hands on the front leg (or floor)
- Eye gaze down to the mat

BENEFITS

- Helps realign spine
- Creates flexibility in the legs and hips
- Relieves stress
- Reduces hunching of shoulders and upper back

MODIFICATIONS

- Bring hands to leg until you can comfortably bring fingertips to floor

PARTNER WITH:
TRIANGLE, LOW LUNGE, TWISTED LUNGE
AND EXTENDED ONE LEG POSE

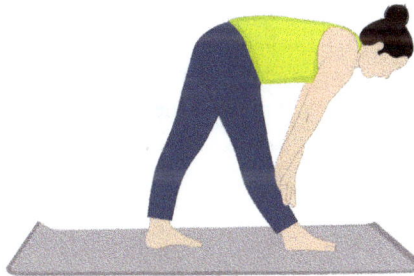

Pyramid Pose

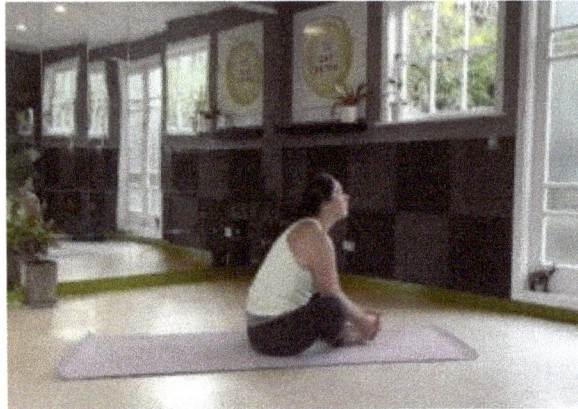

Butterfly Pose
(Badha Konasana)

JOURNEY INWARDS TO CONNECT THE DOTS AND CLOSE
YOUR ENERGITIC CIRCUITS.

STUDIO CUES

- From seated with legs straight in front, drop the feet out to open through the hips
- Bend knees and bring the soles of the feet together
- Sit tall and fold forward from the hips, wrap the hands around the feet
- Use pressure from the elbows into the calves to gently deepen the stretch
- Keep back flat and only drop the head at the end point of the stretch

BENEFITS

- Inner thigh and lower back stretch
- Tones pelvic region
- Calms the mind and aids relaxation
- Relieves menstrual discomfort

MODIFICATIONS

- Place a cushion under the hips to tilt the pelvis forward
- Take time to breath and relax into the pose, don't bounce or push as the muscles will only contract in protest
- Alternatively roll chin down to chest and stretch into the mid-back (kidneys)

PARTNER WITH:
HEAD BEYOND KNEE, BOAT
AND SEATED HALF SPINAL TWIST POSES

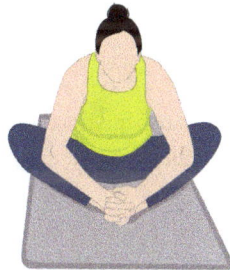

Butterfly Pose

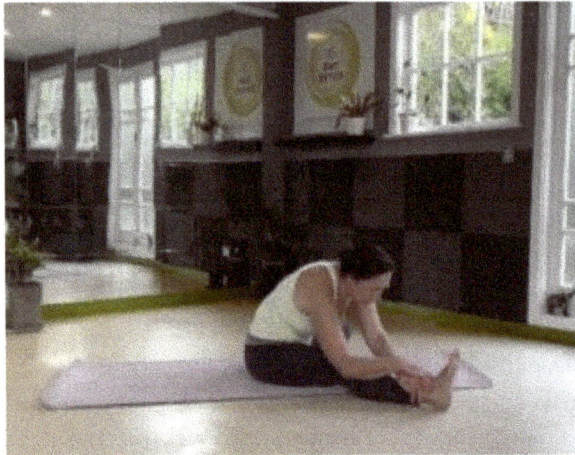

Head Beyond Knee Pose
(Janu Sirsasana)

ACKNOWLEDGE YOUR PRESENT LIMITS TO SEE BEYOND
THE CURRENT SITUATION.

STUDIO CUES
- Start seated with legs comfortably wide
- Bend left knee and place foot on right inner thigh
- Sit forward as you tilt the tailbone back
- Twist the upper body and reach with the opposite hand to foot/leg
- Fold, leading with the chin and chest to maintain a flat back
- Eye gaze to the big toe

BENEFITS

- Deep lower back stretch to reduce pain
- Releases tension in the hip area
- Stimulates digestion
- Improves sleep

MODIFICATIONS

- Most of us will benefit from sitting on the edge of a cushion to tilt the pelvis forward
- If the leg muscles are tight bend the knee and place a cushion under the knee

PARTNER WITH:
BUTTERFLY, BOAT AND SAGE VARIATION POSES

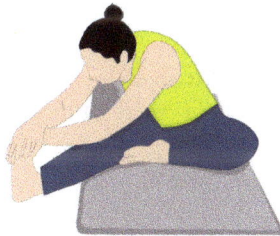

Head Beyond Knee Pose

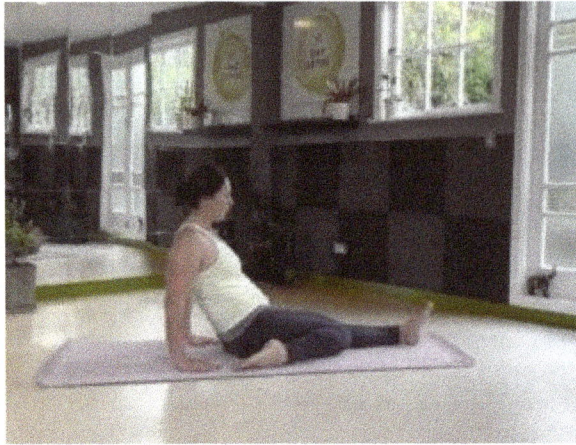

Reclining Half Hero Pose
(Ardha Supta Virasana)

STRETCH YOUR PERSPECTIVE AND TEST NEW PARADIGMS.

STUDIO CUES

- This is not a pose to do if you have any issues with knees, or limited range of motion in the ankles
- Start seated with legs straight ahead, roll to the left and bend the right knee to place the foot beside the right hip
- Foot sits beside the hip with toes pointed, knees remain together
- Place hands on floor behind with fingers forward
- Lean back by bending the elbows to deepen the stretch
- Drop the head at the last to look back (or close your eyes to journey inwards)

BENEFITS

- Front of the thigh (quads) stretch
- Energizes the legs
- Deep stretch for the ankles
- Relieves menopause symptoms

MODIFICATIONS

- Sit on a cushion or yoga block to ease the pressure on the ankle

PARTNER WITH:
BRIDGE, SEATED HALF SPINAL TWIST
AND EXTENDED CHILD'S POSE

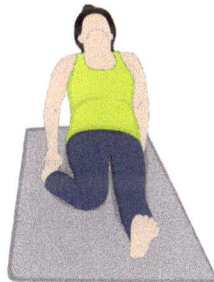

Reclining Half Hero Pose

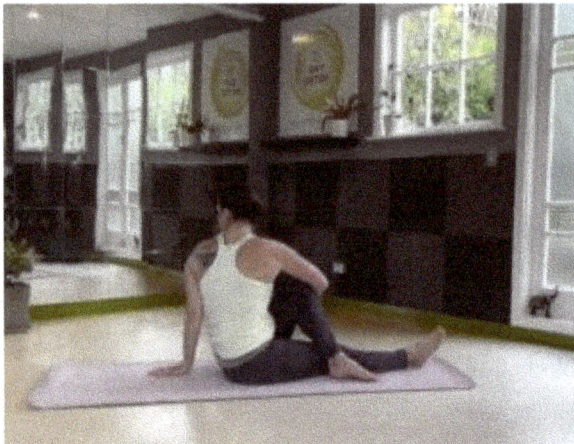

Seated Half Spinal Twist Pose
(Ardha Matsyendrasana)

WRING OUT YOUR BODY TO ARRIVE REFRESHED AND RENEWED.

STUDIO CUES

- Begin seated with legs together and straight
- Bend the right leg and cross it over the left, move the left leg slightly across the mid-line
- Bent leg has foot flat to floor
- Wrap opposite arm around the knee, twist from the core and place the back hand flat to floor
- Look over the shoulder with head neutral and eye gaze softened

BENEFITS

- Wring out the tension all the way down the small muscles along the spine
- Relieves back pain
- Massage for the digestive organs
- Tones reproductive organs
- Extend range of the neck muscles (think looking behind in the car)

MODIFICATIONS

- Place foot on a block if it doesn't reach the floor
- Hold hands to knee for support
- Use a chair to sit upright and reach the opposite hand to knee

PARTNER WITH:
ALL POSES

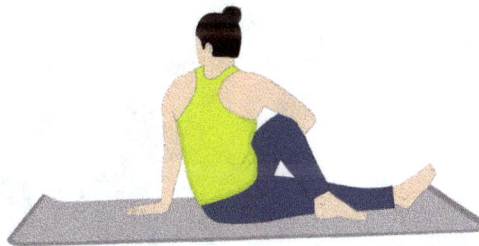

Seated Half Spinal Twist Pose

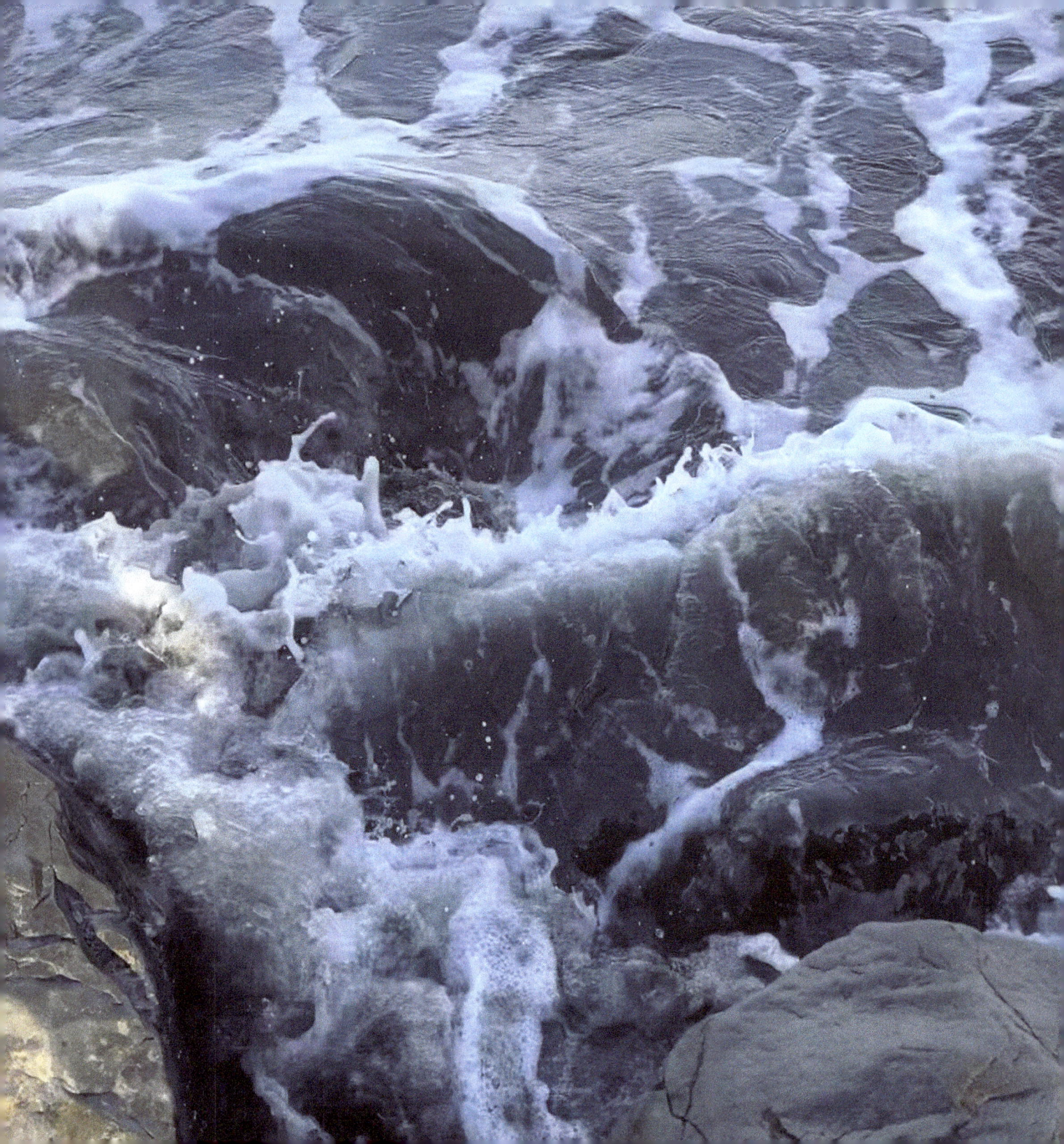

WEEK FOUR - improving Core Strength

Strength in the core is from your hips to your shoulders, both the front of the body as well as the back. When you have core strength you can remain upright without support, you engage the largest muscles closest to your centre rather than the smaller muscles further away. Ever tried to lift something and noticed your neck was doing all the work! Not ideal - more common than you would think - and likely to lead to injury.

Grounded vs Centred: It is possible to be grounded, stable in your environment, but what happens when when the "rug is pulled from beneath the feet", that moment when everything you know to be true is changed in an instant. This is where "centred" will provide the answer. Centred is your inner compass point, the place of stillness in the middle of the washing machine of life.

STUDIO COMMENTS

1. Let the heart rate guide you! It will elevate as you exert yourself. Let it recover with an easy stretch before moving forward to the next activity.

2. A dynamic warmup such as the Sun Salutation sequence helps to prepare the body for the strength poses.

3. Intersperse strength-building poses with releases and stretches for active recovery and balance.

4. Practice with "core engagement". Called "bandha" in Sanskrit, this is an energetic lock. For core strength it can be achieved by - engaging the pelvic floor (pull up as if stopping mid-pee), tuck the tailbone under (lengthen the front of the hips), and pull belly button to spine. This lock will provide stability and protection of the weaker muscles.

5. Early attempts at Week Two's Stability session may have relied on luck (finding the sweet spot). As you develop core strength you will be stronger in the transitions in and out of poses too.

6. The ability to be in Movement (flow), plus the Strength to maintain a pose (hold), develops Endurance (the capacity to sustain a prolonged stressful activity).

PRACTICE SEQUENCE

In this week's gentle flow yoga session let's focus on all things CORE related. You will move from seated to kneeling to lying on both your back and stomach as we activate all the muscles between shoulders and hips. Also, here is a chance to give the legs and hips a break! We deliberately let go of the need to be in constant movement. A slower pace allows for a better understanding of the body's messages.

Begin with a seated version of **Mountain** pose to warm up the shoulders. Come into **Tabletop** and move through the breath coordinated movement of **Cat Cow**. Hold **Plank** for as long as you can maintain good form, then rest in **Extended Child's** pose. Repeat 1-2 times more. As part of the active recovery do the **Wrist Releases**. Come onto the stomach for **Forearm Plank** and **Locust**. Move to seated for **Butterfly** and **Boat**. Lie on the back for **Bridge**. Lastly use **Reclined Spinal Twist** and **Snow Angel** to stretch and release any tension that built up through the efforts.

BALANCE

Have you noticed that some days you have good balance, and other days it's nowhere to be found!

Factors to consider internally are lack of sleep, fatigue and stress. As you build core strength these will have less impact on your state of being. Balance is not a matter of landing the correct position and hoping for the best. Rather a building of the neural pathways that allow a constant readjusting of the body to remain in position - no matter the influences.

Externally we are always being effected by the unseen energies of our environment. Of particular interest to me has been the influence of the moon phases on our physical and emotional bodies. Call it the full moon crazies if you wish. Stories abound of more extreme behaviours around this time. Within the studio it is clear that a couple of days either side of both the new moon and full moon are inherently unstable.

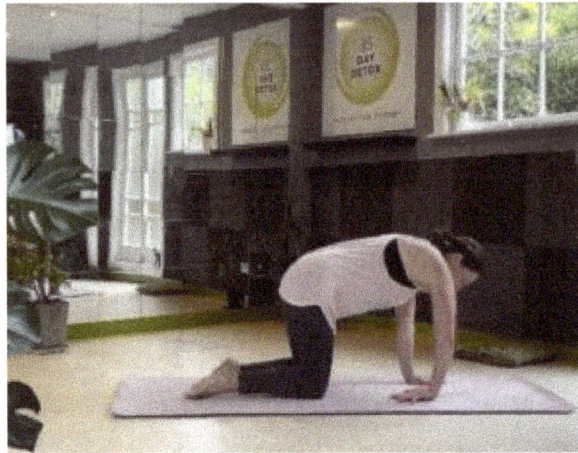

Wrist Releases
(Manibandha Naman)

PRACTICE LETTING GO OF THE NEED TO CONTROL ALL
THE DETAILS OF YOUR LIFE.

STUDIO CUES

- Be very mindful of small muscles, ligaments and bones and go gently
- Once the hand is in position deepen the stretch by carefully straightening the arm
- Begin in **Tabletop** taking care to place the hands under the shoulders each time
- Turn hands so fingertips point out to the edge of the mat, release and return to **Tabletop** for recovery
- Next turn hands so fingers point inwards to each other
- Next turn hands so fingers point back to the knees
- Lastly, turn the hands palm-up and place the backs of the hands on the floor under the shoulders, all the way to the wrist crease

BENEFITS

- Counters stiffness from repetitive actions
- Wrist strength will absorb some of the impact if you trip, important as we age healthily
- Develop strength in the wrists to support body weight-bearing yoga poses

MODIFICATIONS

- Do one hand at a time to use the other hand for support

PARTNER WITH:
PLANK, COBRA AND KNEELING SUPERMAN POSES

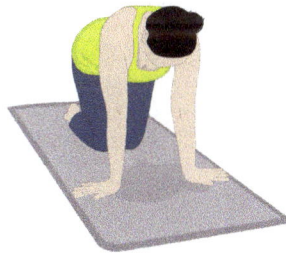

Wrist Releases

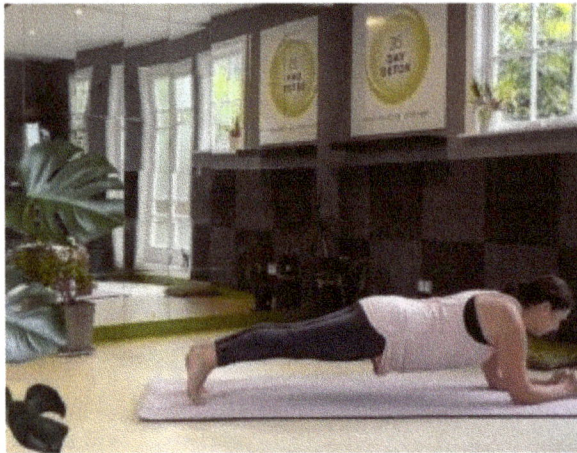

Forearm Plank Pose
(Modified Phalakasana)

A STATE OF GRACE COMES FROM KNOWING YOU HAVE PUT
THE REQUIRED EFFORT IN.

STUDIO CUES

- Begin lying on the stomach with elbows under shoulders and palms on the mat shoulder width apart
- Tuck toes under and push heels back to lift the knees
- Engage legs by pulling kneecaps up
- Push through the elbows to lift the hips
- Drop hips into line with shoulders and pull belly button to spine
- Maintain a neutral neck and eye gaze down to the mat, relax the hands

BENEFITS

- Builds core strength without loading the wrists
- Great antidote to sitting for extended periods
- Energizes the body and mind

MODIFICATIONS

- It is better to drop to the knees and maintain a strong plank than suffer unnecessarily
- Multiple sets of 3-5 breaths are as effective as one long hold

PARTNER WITH:
EXTENDED CHILD'S POSE, THREAD THE NEEDLE AND
KNEELING HIP RELEASES

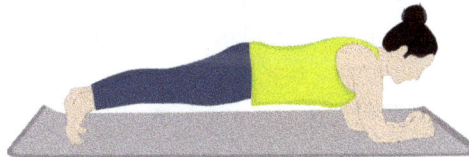

Forearm Plank Pose

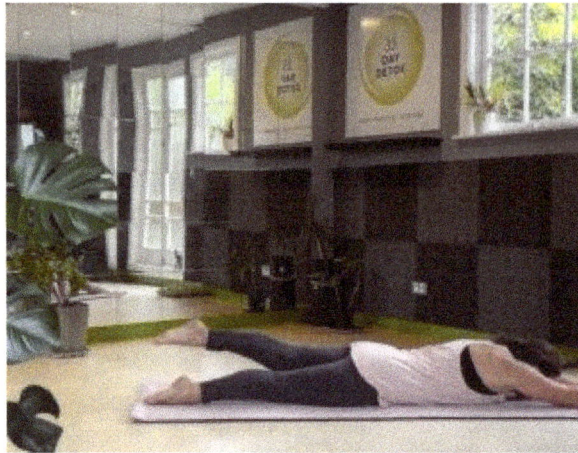

Locust Pose
(Salabhasana)

CONSIDER THE RESOURCES ALREADY AVAILABLE TO YOU.
THE SUPPORT YOU NEED LIES READY.

STUDIO CUES

- Lie on the stomach with arms extended in front, palms on the floor
- Rest chin on the floor
- Arms are shoulder width apart, feet are flat to the floor and hip width apart
- Pull ankles towards each other to stop feet and hips rolling out
- Lift right leg and left arm as high as comfortable, without bending either
- Toes are pointed and palms are facing down
- Lift chin from floor if it's OK on the neck

BENEFITS

- Strengthen lower back muscles
- Improves breathing
- Strengthen pelvic area
- Stimulate reproductive organs

MODIFICATIONS

- Lift the same arm and leg for 3-5 breaths, swap to the other side
- Lift both arms and legs plus chin for the full expression of the pose

PARTNER WITH:
CAT COW AND EXTENDED CHILD'S POSE

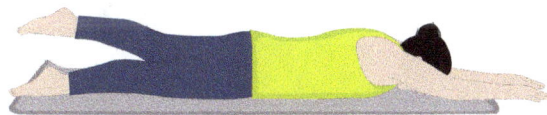

Locust Pose

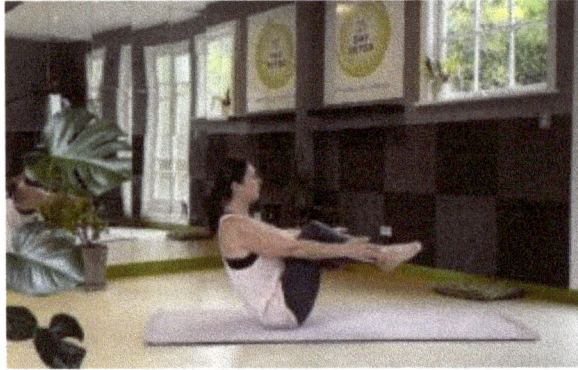

Boat Pose
(Navasana)

HOLDING STEADFAST IN THE ROCKY TIMES WILL TAKE
YOU TO A NEW PLACE.

STUDIO CUES

- Start seated, knees bent, feet on the floor and hands lightly on knees
- Find the balance point on the buttocks
- Lift feet to knee height
- Lift the chin and chest to maintain spinal integrity (avoid strain/injury to the lower back)
- Release hands from legs and stretch them forward with straight arms
- Eye gaze passed the toes, and breathe!

BENEFITS

- Builds confidence
- Reduces stress
- Tones abdominal muscles
- Stimulates reproductive organs
- Strengthens hip flexor muscles

MODIFICATIONS

- Start by lifting one leg at a time to engage the hip flexors
- Multiple sets of 3-5 breaths are more effective than one long hold where alignment is compromised
- Adjust to seated in a chair by lifting the leg and straightening for 3-5 breaths

PARTNER WITH:
BUTTERFLY, SAGE VARIATION
AND HEAD BEYOND KNEE POSES

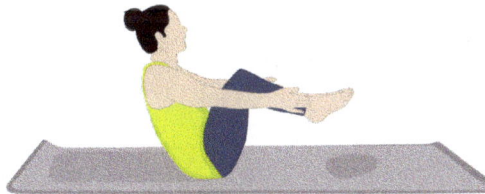

Boat Pose

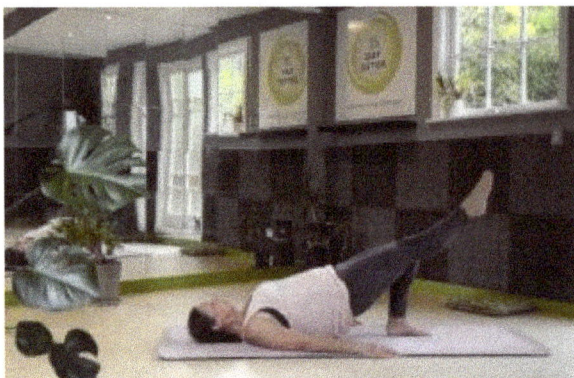

Bridge Pose
(Setu Bandhasana)

STRENGTH WITHIN STILLNESS ALLOWS YOU TO SEE THE WAY FORWARD.

STUDIO CUES

- Lie on back with knees bent and feet as close to buttocks as comfortable
- Feet hip width apart or closer together for the single leg variation
- Push heels into the ground to raise the hips
- Relax the gluteal muscles to activate the hamstring muscles
- Hands on the floor for support only
- Single leg variation has knees together
- Eye gaze to the ceiling (or eyes closed), and breathe

BENEFITS

- Strengthens hamstrings
- Improves digestion
- Stimulates the lymphatic system
- Works to balance the hormonal system

MODIFICATIONS

- Multiple short holds will build strength without cramping the hamstrings

PARTNER WITH:
KNEELING HIP RELEASES AND RECLINED SPINAL TWIST POSES

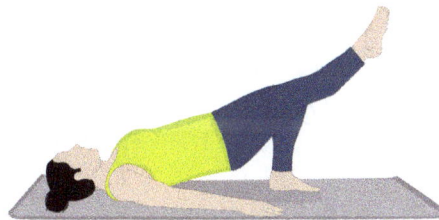

Bridge Pose

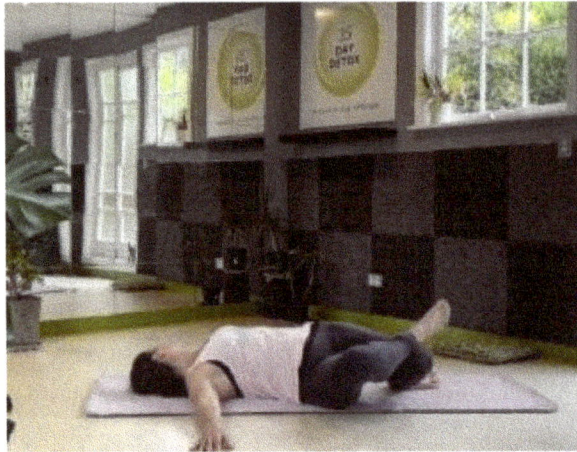

Reclined Spinal Twist Pose
(Supta Matsyendrasana)

REGULARLY RELEASE THE PRESSURE VALVES TO DISPERSE
EXCESS ENERGY FROM THE BODY.

STUDIO CUES

- Lie on back with knees bent and feet hip width apart
- Place right foot on the top of the left knee
- Arms on the floor, palms down, at shoulder height for support
- Drop knees to the right, using the weight of the top foot to gently deepen the stretch
- Have the hip and knee equally away from the floor
- Look over the left shoulder to the left middle finger (or eyes can close as you drop your awareness inwards)

BENEFITS

- Relieves tension in the lower back
- Calms the nervous system
- Aids lymphatic drainage

MODIFICATIONS

- Keep both feet on the floor for an easier twist
- Lie on the bed for a gentle full body twist and stretch

PARTNER WITH:
BOAT, BRIDGE AND SNOW ANGEL POSES

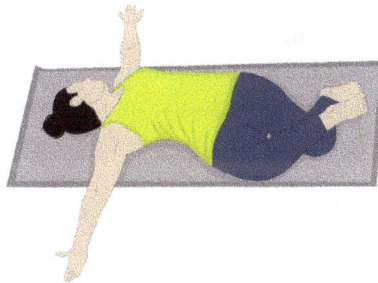

Reclined Spinal Twist Pose

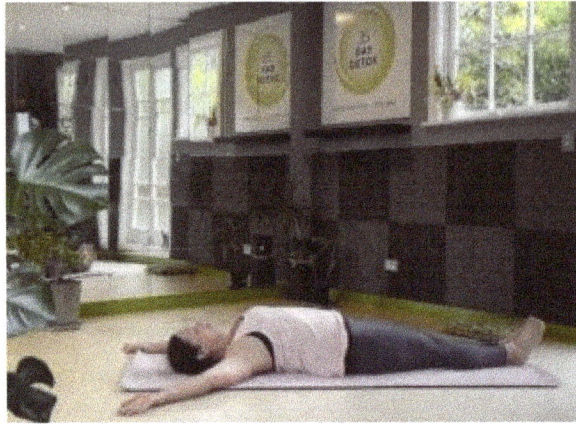

Snow Angel Pose
(Savasana variation)

SURRENDER TO WHAT IS. ACCEPTANCE IS THE KEY TO
MOVING FORWARD.

STUDIO CUES

- Begin by lying on your back with legs relaxed
- Arms are beside the hips with palms facing up
- Ensure the body is aligned and head neutral
- Keep all points (fingers, wrists, elbows and shoulders) on the floor as you slowly sweep the arms out and up
- Take the time to stop and breathe before moving further into the pose

BENEFITS

- Counters time spent hunched over computers or driving
- Front of shoulder and chest release
- Improves lung capacity by stretching the chest muscles
- Calms the mind

MODIFICATIONS

- Immediately come out of the stretch is there is any nerve tingling or numbness in the hands
- Lie on the bed to stretch and focus on long slow breathing

PARTNER WITH:
HAPPY BABY AND RECLINED SPINAL TWIST POSES

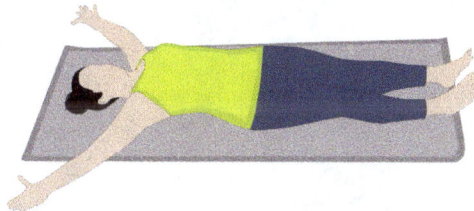

Snow Angel Pose

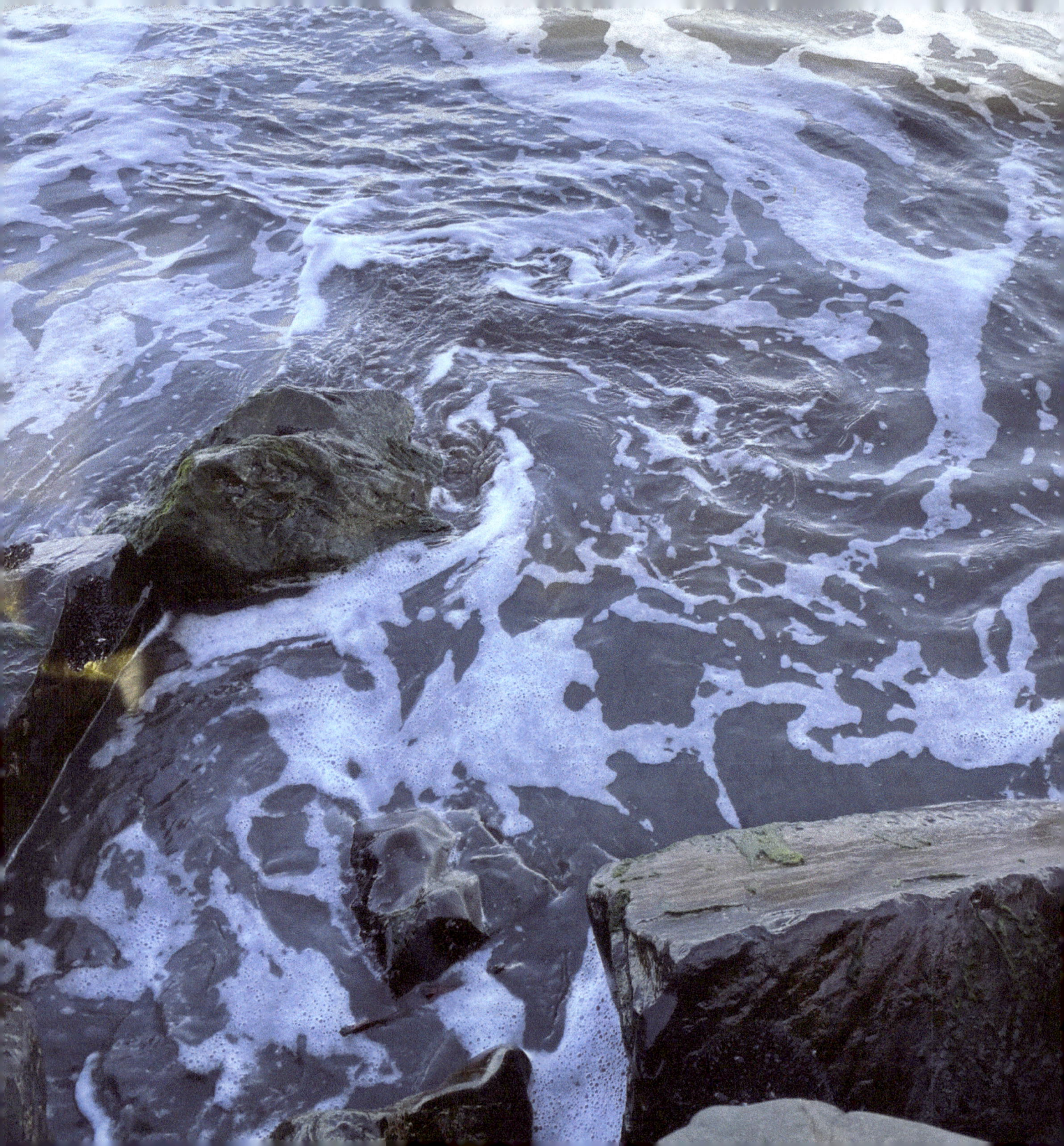

WEEK FIVE - strengthen Upper Body

Having first created a sense of stability and balance, we moved to build the foundations by stretching and strengthening the hips and legs. Next we improved our ability to withstand situations with core strength. Now you are ready to express yourself with this upper body strength and release sequence. As we extend our arms we expand our sphere of influence. No longer being prepared to play it small!

Grief is about coming into the acceptance of loss. Loss in all it's forms - loved ones, jobs, relationships, financial, and opportunities. A strong sense of who you really are is required, reconnecting to that person before life took all it's twists and turns. Then comes the discipline of showing up regardless of the current situation. Only when we accept where were are at can we move forward.

STUDIO COMMENTS

1. As you stretch more frequently and deeper, cramps (especially in the feet when working with the upper body) are common. Proving the point that nothing within us is disconnected. Please consult your medical practitioner if they persist.

2. Consider your daily yoga practice as a game of two halves. The first half is a more active and dynamic flow. This is where all the challenging work is done. The second half is where you come down closer to the mat and do the deeper slower stretches that create the changes you are looking for in your body and mind.

3. Breath and movement is a natural part of improving the lung capacity. Practice the "one breath - one movement" of this gentle flow yoga. If in doubt as to whether it is an inhale or exhale then this guide works well - inhale as you move arms/legs away from the heart and exhale as you bring arms/legs back to the heart centre.

4. Mastery of the gentle yoga flow comes from the understanding that the transition from one pose to another is as important as the poses themselves.

PRACTICE SEQUENCE

This gentle flow yoga session is designed to build strength and flexibility in the upper body. Feel like you have the weight of the world on your shoulders? Use these poses to release the tension!

Often we are focused on the lower body and the upper body is neglected. Yet this is where the tension headaches can stem from. And building strength can go a long way to relieving chronic tension. This week's poses will also stretch out the front, back and sides of the body too.

Start kneeling, sitting back on the heels to create pressure between the calves and hamstrings, stimulating blood flow. Move forward to **Tabletop** pose and pause to release tension in the spine and warmup the shoulders with **Cat Cow**. Walk the hands forward and sink the forward to the floor in **Puppy** for 3-5 breaths. Lift the head and walk the hands back to come up to the knees. Turn lengthways on the mat and come into **Gate**. Return to kneeling and tuck the toes and lift the hips into **Downdog** for 3-5 breaths. Walk hands to feet and rest in **Forward Fold**. Walk hands forward again and this time lift the right leg and twist the body for **Wild Thing**. Repeat for the other side. Take your time and come to the front of the mat - standing with hands in prayer. Step back to **Triangle**, switch the feet position to do the other side. Step forward and come into the stillness of **Eagle**. On your way to finish, stop briefly in seated to stretch the shoulders with the **Sage Variation**. Lastly rest and reflect in **Reclined Butterfly**.

YOGA TO DETOXIFY

Your yoga practice is a detoxification process. At a physical level, increasing blood flow throughout the entire body and stimulating the lymphatic system. These two systems (active and passive) work together to aid in clearing dead cells from the body. At an emotional level, where you tap into the store cupboard of unprocessed experiences. The stimulation (stretching and squeezing) action helps in the release of long held tension. At a mental level, where you make new shapes and hold positions to go beyond what you previously thought was possible. The breath ties the physical, emotional and mental bodies together.

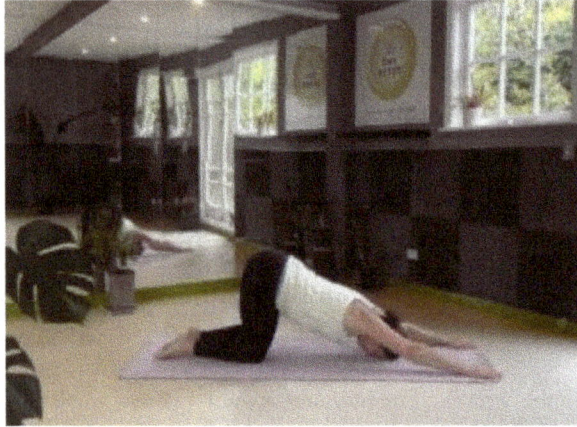

Puppy Pose
(Uttana Shishosana)

BOW IN GRATITUDE FOR WHAT IS GOOD IN LIFE. GATHER STRENGTH TO CHANGE WHAT IS NOT.

STUDIO CUES

- Start by kneeling in **Tabletop**, ensure the hips remain over the knees
- Tops of feet are flat to the floor to deepen the stretch throughout the body
- Engage the core to protect the lower back
- Forehead to floor, or a cushion or yoga block
- Elbows straight and fingers stretched wide to deepen the stretch under the arms and chest

BENEFITS

- Calms the mind
- Stretches under arms and chest muscles
- Realigns and lengthens the back

MODIFICATIONS

- Bend elbows and place them on the mat to soften the upper body stretch

PARTNER WITH:
THREAD THE NEEDLE AND CAT COW POSES

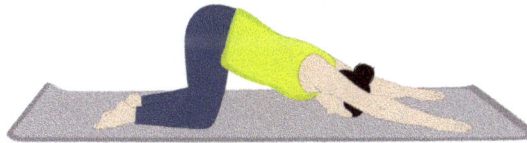

Puppy Pose

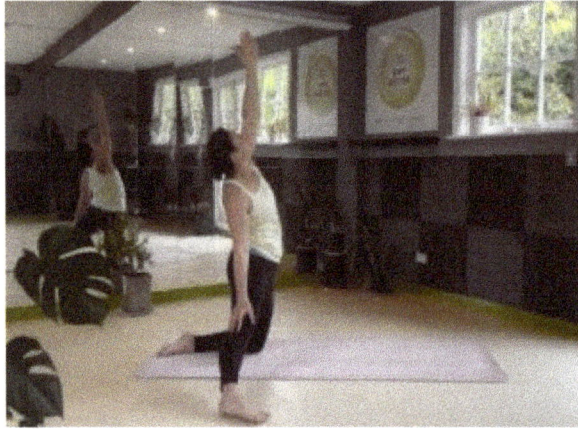

Gate Pose
(Parighasana)

REACH OUT OF THE SMALLNESS OF LIFE AND EXPAND
INTO ITS POTENTIAL.

STUDIO CUES

- Begin on knees
- Raise the left arm making sure the left side is all in one line - wrist over shoulder, over hip, over knee
- Engage the core
- Reach tall and push the hips slightly forward
- Deepen the stretch by bending the right elbow and allowing the left arm to go beyond the crown of the head

BENEFITS

- Energise the whole body
- Activates the major chakra points
- Stimulate digestion
- Calms a stress response

MODIFICATIONS

- Place a cushion under the knee
- If shoulder mobility is an issue keep the hand on the hip rather than raising it overhead
- Eyes remain focused straight ahead if you experience any vertigo or dizziness

PARTNER WITH:
RECLINING HALF HERO POSE

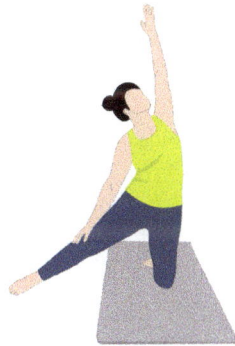

Gate Pose

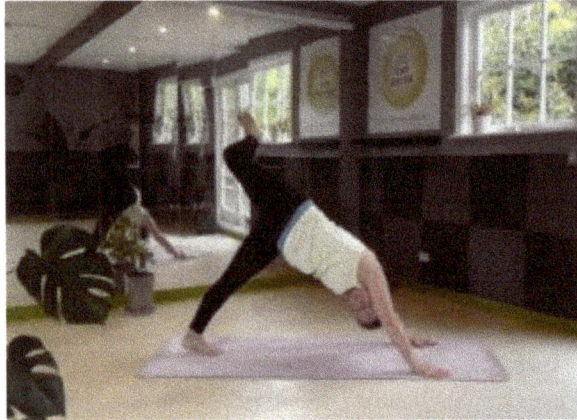

Wild Thing Pose
(Camatkarasana)

SURPISE AND DELIGHT WITH THE UNEXPECTED TWISTS
LIFE BRINGS.

STUDIO CUES

- Begin in **Downdog** and raise the right leg so that it is line with the spine
- Flex the foot and bend the knee
- Twist from the hips to stack one hip above the other
- Look under the armpit (stay here to build upper body strength)

BENEFITS

- Stretch through the front of the body
- Build strength in the upper body
- Tones reproductive organs
- Develop trust and confidence to go beyond that which you can see
- Sparks joy and lightness of being

MODIFICATIONS

- As you build confidence it is possible to drop the foot to the floor for the full expression of the pose

PARTNER WITH:
DOWNDOG AND TWISTED LUNGE POSES

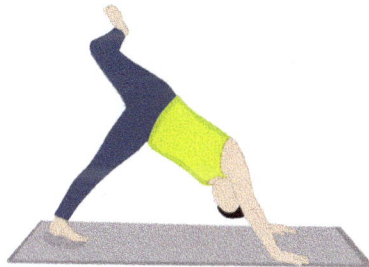

Wild Thing Pose

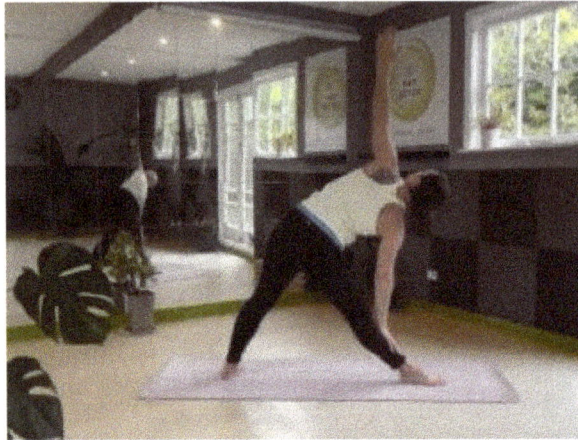

Triangle Pose
(Trikonasana)

CLAIM ALL THE YOU ARE.

STUDIO CUES

- Start with hands on hips and feet hip width apart
- Step the left foot back with foot facing the side of the mat
- Turn hips back to front of the mat, pull both kneecaps up to straighten your legs
- Engage core as you bring the right hand onto the right leg
- Raise left arm directly above the right in one line stacking the shoulders
- Look up to the thumb if it is OK on the neck

BENEFITS

- Improves stability and focus
- Strengthens legs, hips and core
- Deep stretch through all planes of the body for the legs, hips and back, chest, shoulders and arms
- Expands your horizons

MODIFICATIONS

- Come up safely by looking down first to take the neck off it's stretch, then bring the left hand to hip once more, and rise back up with both hands to hips
- Swap feet positions and repeat on the other side
- If balance is an issue remain with the eye gaze down to the mat (or neutral to the wall)
- Take the pressure off the shoulder by remaining with hand to hip

PARTNER WITH:
STANDING SIDE STRETCHES AND PYRAMID POSES

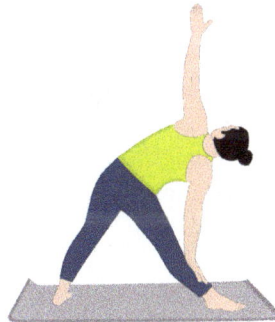

Triangle Pose

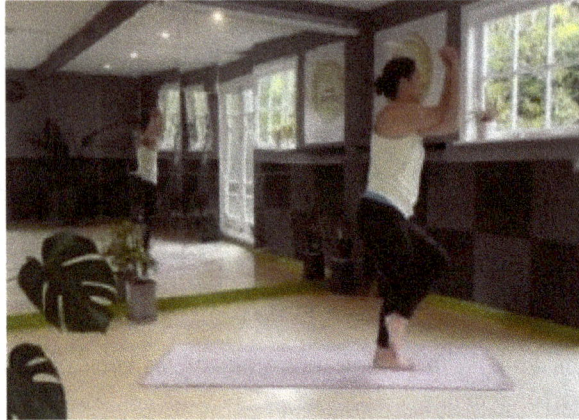

Eagle Pose
(Garudasana)

GUARD YOUR POTENTIAL CLOSE TO THE HEART BEFORE
ALLOWING IT FREEDOM TO FLY.

STUDIO CUES

- Start with hands on hips to keep them straight
- Bend at the ankle and the knee of the standing (left) leg
- Place opposite (right) leg over as if sitting and crossing the legs at the knees
- Wrap arms the opposite way to legs (left over right), crossing at the elbows
- Hold hands together, deepen the stretch by lifting the elbows and moving the hands away from the face
- Focus eyes through the space between the forearms

BENEFITS

- Strengthen ankles and knees
- Improves balance and focus
- Deep stretch for the shoulders
- Builds connection between the mind and the body
- Calls time on over-thinking

MODIFICATIONS

- Keep the toes on the floor until you can maintain good balance
- If arms can't cross then bring palms of the hands together, bend elbows and bring elbows to touch
- Practice the arm position seated on the floor or in a chair

PARTNER WITH:
MOUNTAIN AND PYRAMID POSES

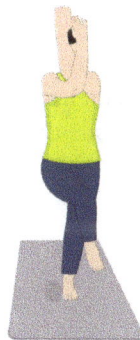

Eagle Pose

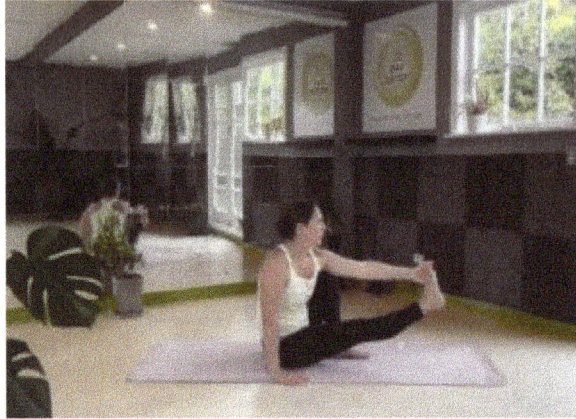

Sage Variation Pose (Marichyasana variation)

MASTER THE PHYSICAL BODY TO ACCESS THE NON-PHYSICAL REALMS.

STUDIO CUES

- Start seated with legs straight, hands on the floor for support
- Bend the left leg and bring the left foot close the the body
- Bend the right leg to reach for the right foot with the left hand
- Push the foot into the hand to create the shoulder stretch

BENEFITS

- Use your body to safely stretch in the shoulder
- Improves posture
- Releases tension in the shoulder and neck
- Stimulates lymphatic system

MODIFICATIONS

- Use a strap or towel wrapped around the foot if it is difficult to reach

PARTNER WITH:
HEAD BEYOND KNEE AND BOAT POSES

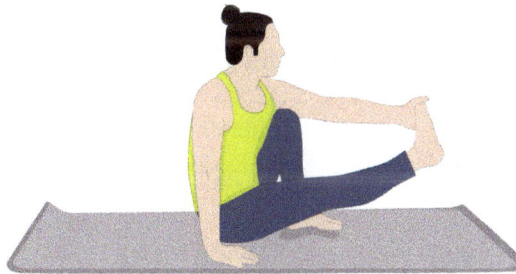

Sage Variation Pose

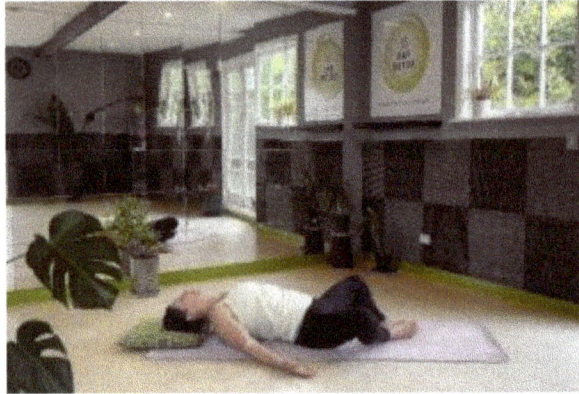

Reclined Butterfly Pose
(Supta Badha Konasana)

PRESENCE IS THE AWARENESS OF SPACE BETWEEN THE BREATH.

STUDIO CUES

- Begin lying on your back (you can use a yoga block/book to deepen the stretch)
- Roll slightly to the side and place the block on the upper back
- Lie back on the block, use a cushion under the head if it doesn't reach the mat
- Roll shoulders open and arms are relaxed and on the floor so that palms face up
- Relax the legs, bend knees and place soles of the feet together
- Take the time after this pose to lie directly on the floor and ensure the natural curve is in the spine

BENEFITS

- Stretch shoulders and inner thighs
- With the use of the block it also stretches across the front of the chest
- Improves breathing
- Relaxes the digestive system
- Helps regulate and balance hormones
- Counters the hunching over from computers, phones and driving
- Relieves sciatic pain

MODIFICATIONS

- If this pose causes pressure around the lower back (sacrum), consider bringing knees together and feet wide, to create more space around the lower spine
- Alternatively place hands on the stomach, ribs or hips - with elbows remaining on the floor for support
- Lie on the bed to nurture and restore your sense of self

PARTNER WITH:
RECLINED SPINAL TWIST AND SNOW ANGEL POSES

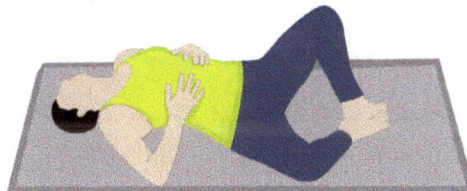

Reclined Butterfly Pose

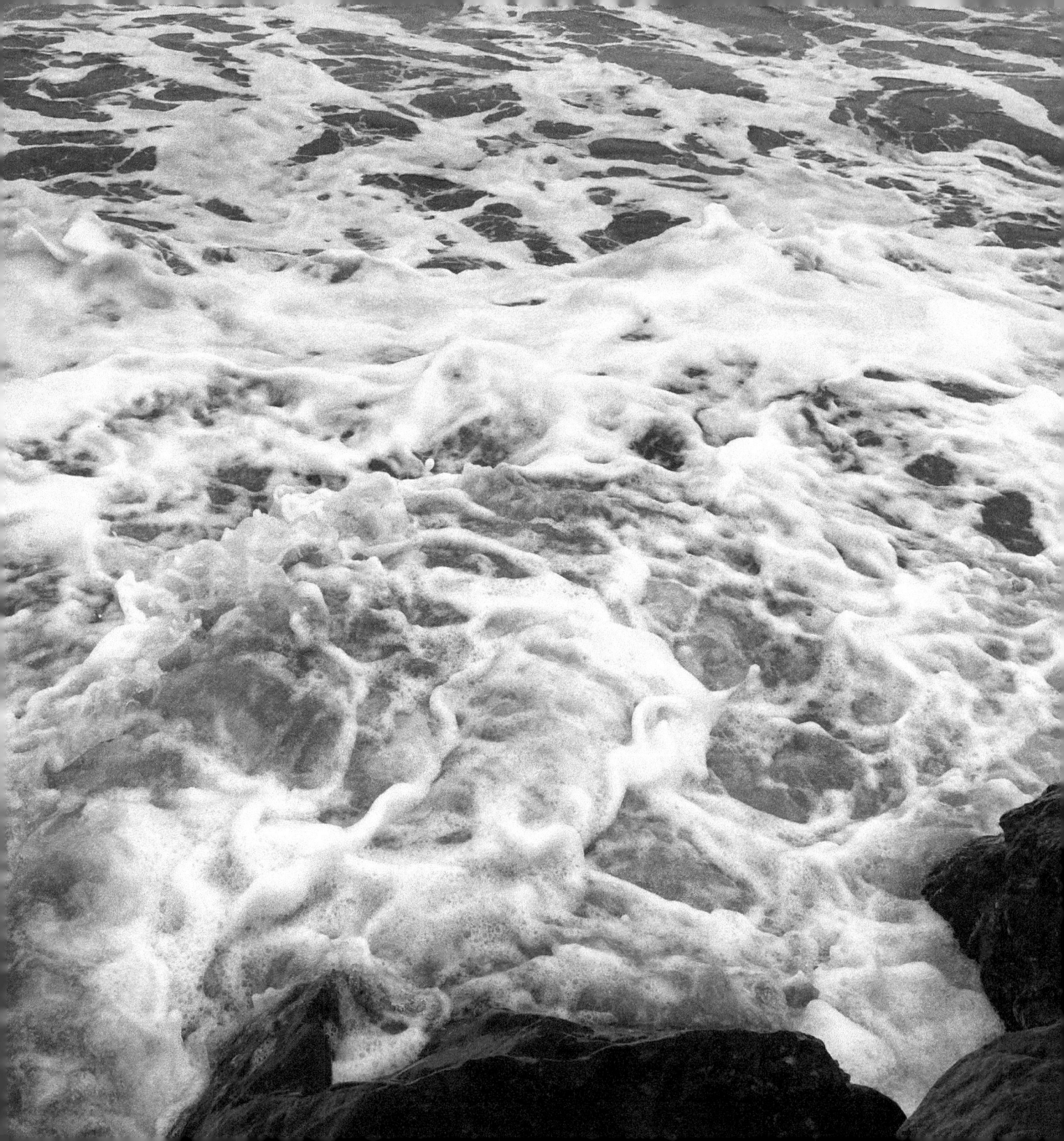

WEEK SIX - a Rest and Recovery session

This week's session may seem easy but it is deceptively powerful. Here you are learning the concept of "one breath with one movement". That there is not a rush to the end - or any sense of achievement needed. We learn to slow down and connect body with breath with mind. To become present in the moment.

The Buddhist saying is that if you don't have time to meditate for 10 minutes per day - then you need to do 20 minutes practice. Most of us do not have a "mission critical" role in life that suggests we need to outsource the mundane and repetitive. Yet we do, and those activities, sweeping the drive, folding the washing, or preparing a meal, can be the most satisfying and calming rituals to add back into your life. Balance is the key to harmony!

STUDIO COMMENTS

1. When even standing can seem an effort - don't let that stop you from doing your daily yoga practice. Start lower to the ground - and as the energy builds you may feel inclined to come up into the standing poses.

2. Take a moment to notice the difference between the side you have worked and the one yet to to do. This provides valuable feedback as to how you are transforming your physical being.

3. Understand the energy lines of your body (vertical, horizontal and diagonal). Visualise the dimensions of the space that you occupy in each direction.

4. Yoga is always working at an energetic level to realign body, mind, and soul with spirit.

5. Recognise the difference between tiredness and exhaustion. You can be tired from the day and a good night's sleep will refresh you ready for the new day. However a good night's sleep will not reset exhaustion. More self-care is needed and yoga can help!

6. Sometimes we get triggered by a situation and the emotional response can be palatable. Then the over-thinking kicks in - and if we don't stop in time - it will lead to overwhelm. Halt this spiral and bring you back into a centred and empowered mindset.

TENSION

Release pent-up tension through the extremities: Shake out the fingers and wrist to relax the shoulders. Wiggle the toes and ankles to release tightness in the hips. And unclench the jaw to relieve the pressure of overthinking.

PRACTICE SEQUENCE

The primary objective of this session is the unblocking energies. Even though we can't see them - these energy sub-stations (chakras) are playing a major role in your current state of mind. As you stimulate (stretch and squeeze) they release heaviness and a lightness comes over the body.

Start down on the ground in **Extended Child's with Side Stretches** pose for 3-5 breaths in each position. Make your way up to **Tabletop** for **Kneeling Hip Releases**, followed by **Cat Cow**, and **Thread the Needle**. Take your time in each pose breathing deeply into the releases possible with the placing of the body into the various shapes. Next challenge yourself with the strength of **Tiger** or **Kneeling Superman**. With the newly gathered energy come up to standing and the **Extended One Leg**, moving the ankles to release tension in the joints. Return to the mat and lie on your back for reclined **Mountain** (overhead stretches). Bring the legs up into **Happy Baby** and rock side-to-side to massage out the the lower back muscles. Lastly come to a comfortable seated position for the **Neck Releases**.

BREATHING TO SUPPORT YOGA FLOW

Use different styles of breathing to achieve different outcomes. Mindful breathing is an important part of the yoga flow. Breathe in and out through the nose to energise and build heat (this will support the detoxification process). After the effort of a sequence or a strength pose, take a breath in through the nose and sigh out through the mouth, to release the tension and any emotional response.

Practice making the breath the same length as the movement. Start the inhale/exhale as you begin to move into a pose and finish the breath as you come into stillness in the expression of the pose. As your lung capacity improves you will notice more time to make the subtle adjustments that reflect your mastery of the present moment.

Above all notice when you have lost connection to the breath, that is the cue to stop and place yourself in one of the recovery poses. Take the time there to connect with what is happening with the mind-space. Thoughts such as - I haven't got time for this, it's too hard, or a rerun of a conversation or situation, are gold for understanding where you are right now.

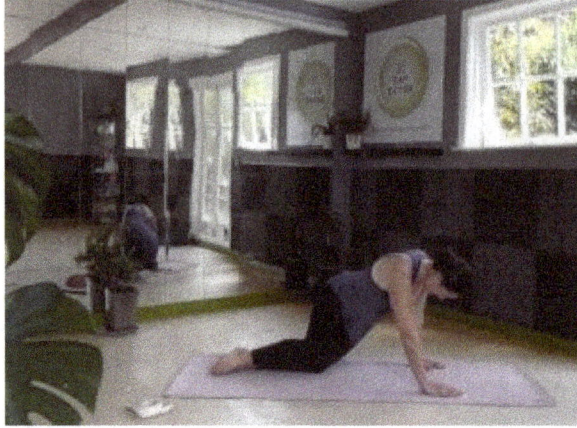

Kneeling Hip Releases (Bharmanasana variation)

CALL TIME ON LONG HELD EMOTIONS. MOVE TO CREATE
A LIGHTNESS OF BEING.

STUDIO CUES

- Start in **Tabletop** pose, bring knees together
- Circle hips clockwise for 3-5 times
- Pause and then circle anticlockwise for the same number, this time with slightly smaller circles
- Keep arms straight

BENEFITS

- Release tension in the hips, lower back and IT Bands
- Stimulate digestion (first moving the large intestine and then the small intestine)
- Build shoulder strength

MODIFICATIONS

- Place a cushion under the knees if they are pressure sensitive
- Make the circles as large or small as comfortable, notice where you pull back from tightness
- Skip this pose if you have had knee surgery

PARTNER WITH:
CAT COW AND EXTENDED CHILD'S POSE

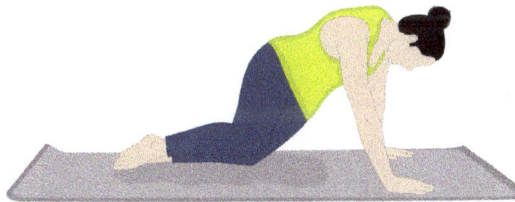

Kneeling Hip Releases

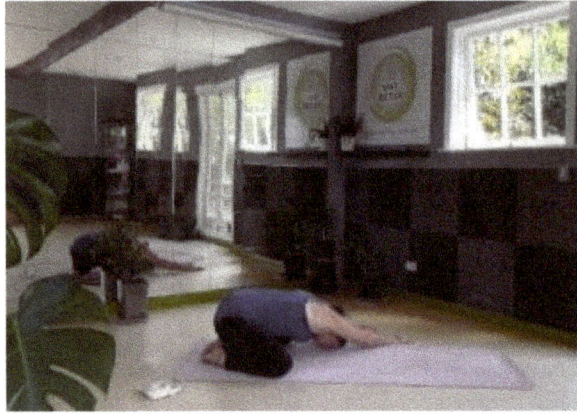

Extended Child's Pose with Side Stretches
(Utthita Balasana variation)

BE OPEN TO NEW POSSIBILITIES.

STUDIO CUES

- Kneel with toes together and knees wide
- Push buttocks back and hands forward
- Walk hands to the right first
- Forehead to floor and arms straight
- Sink hips back to lengthen lower back
- Close your eyes and breathe into the stretch from hip to wrist

BENEFITS

- Stimulates digestion
- Releases tension in the hips

MODIFICATIONS

- Bend the supporting arm and make a fist to support the head if necessary

PARTNER WITH:
LOCUST, KNEELING SUPERMAN AND TIGER POSES

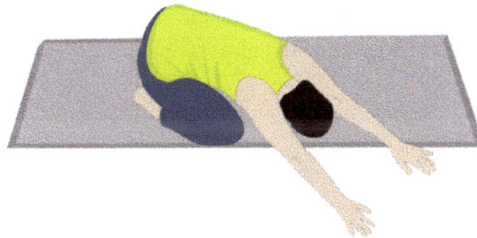

Extended Child's Pose with Side Stretches

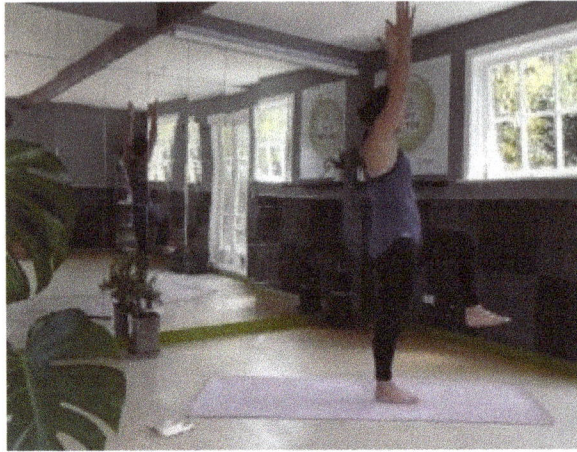

Extended One Leg Pose
(Utthita Ekapadasana)

EMBRACE THE PRESENT MOMENT.

STUDIO CUES

- Start standing with feet hip width apart
- Transfer weight to the left foot, bend the knee and raise it to hip height, ankle is directly under the knee
- Ensure the standing leg is strong with foot pushing into floor and kneecap pulled up
- Belly button to spine to lift the leg from the core muscles
- Raise arms overhead, shoulder width apart, with palms facing in

BENEFITS

- Strengthen leg and hip
- Clear the mind of unwanted thoughts

MODIFICATIONS

- Keep hands on hips until the strength and balance is further developed
- With hands on hips practice circling out the ankles in one direction and then the other
- Straighten the raised leg and point and flex the ankle 3-5 times

PARTNER WITH:
MOUNTAIN, PYRAMID AND TRIANGLE POSES

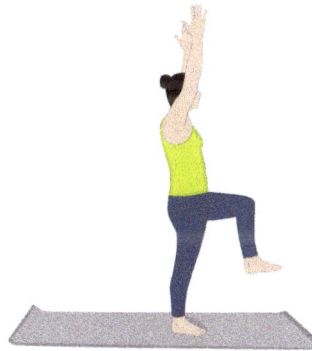

Extended One Leg Pose

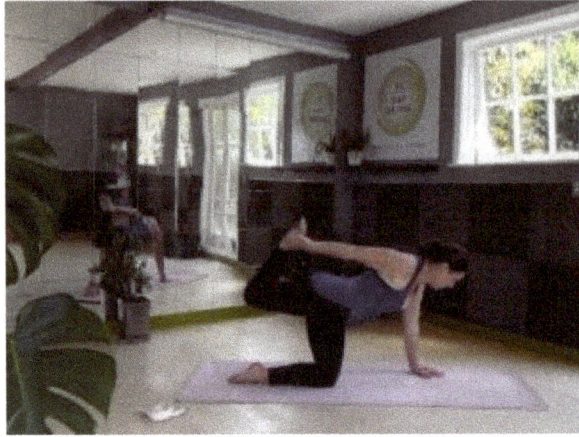

Tiger Pose
(Vyaghrasana)

CONFIDENCE IS THE KEY. TRUST AND FAITH WILL TAKE YOU FURTHER.

STUDIO CUES

- Start in **Tabletop** pose, bring knees and hands a little closer for extra balance
- Raise the right leg to hip height, bend the knee and flex the foot
- Stretch the left arm forward to create extra space in the shoulder
- Sweep the arm around to reach the right leg, move the hand to hold the right ankle and flex the foot
- Eye gaze directly down to the mat

BENEFITS

- Stretch the quad muscles
- Strengthen the core
- Steady the mind
- Let go of an over-thinking mind

MODIFICATIONS

- Place a cushion under the knee if it is pressure sensitive
- Use a belt or towel wrapped around the ankle if you can't reach the leg yet

PARTNER WITH:
CAT COW AND DOWNDOG POSES

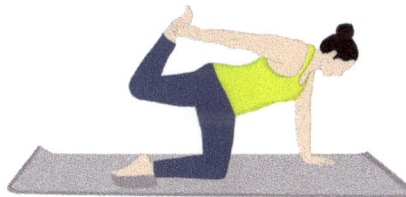

Tiger Pose

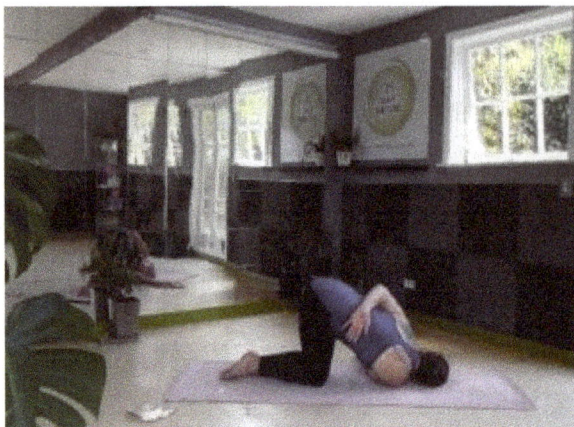

Thread the Needle Pose
(Urdhva Mukha Pasasana)

UNLOCK JOY WITHIN AND COMPASSION FOR OTHERS.

STUDIO CUES

- Start in **Tabletop** pose and slide right arm through between the left leg and arm, palm facing up
- Right ear and right shoulder rest on the floor
- Lengthen through the spine by stretching the toes flat to the floor
- Focus the eyes on the resting middle finger of the (right) hand

BENEFITS

- Releases tension in the neck
- Stretches the upper back muscles
- Works to realign the spinal muscles
- Counters the effects of frozen shoulder

MODIFICATIONS

- Use a yoga block or cushion if the head doesn't comfortably reach the floor
- Once the head is on the floor you can deepen the pose by placing the left hand on the mid-back
- If Vertigo is an issue then **Sage Variation** may be a better option

PARTNER WITH:
CAT COW AND PUPPY POSES

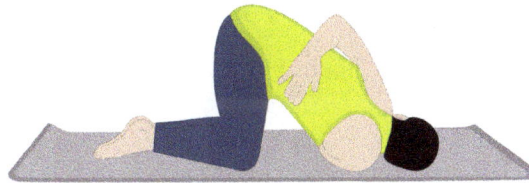

Thread the Needle Pose

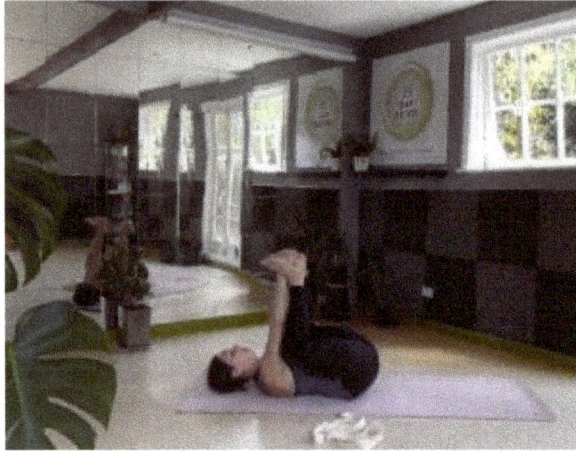

Happy Baby Pose
(Ananda Balasana)

WE CAN CHOOSE TO ROCK OUR OWN BOAT.

STUDIO CUES

- Lie on back with head on the floor and knees bent
- Lift the feet above the hips with knees bent and reach each hand for the instep of the corresponding foot
- Knees track out towards the armpits and soles of the feet face up to the sky
- Head and tailbone remain on the floor
- Gently rock side to side to use the weight of the body to massage the lower back muscles

BENEFITS

- Relaxing and calming
- Brings joy to the mat

MODIFICATIONS

- Start with **Half Happy Baby -** left leg bent with foot on the floor, raise right leg and reach for the right foot with the right hand, left hand on the floor for support
- Hold the back of the corresponding leg if you cannot reach the foot yet
- Lie on the bed to reduce pressure on the spine

PARTNER WITH:
BRIDGE AND RECLINED SPINAL TWIST POSES

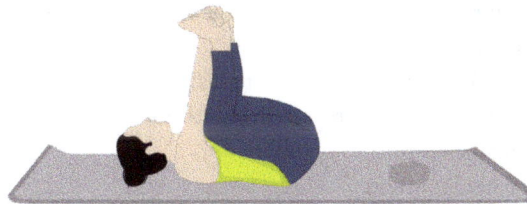

Happy Baby Pose

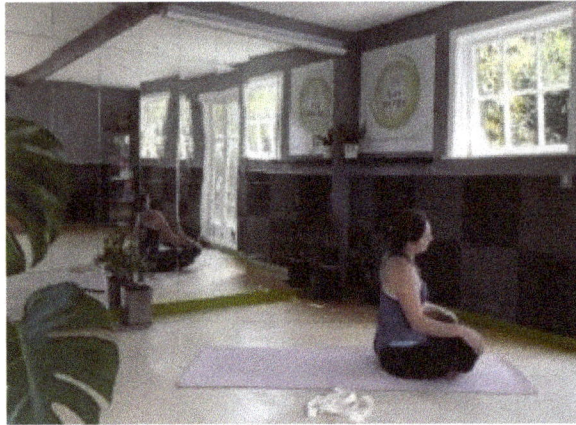

Neck Releases
(Sukhasana variation)

BE CLEAR AND HONEST WITH YOURSELF ABOUT YOUR
CURRENT SITUATION AND WHAT YOUR PURPOSE FOR
BEING IS.

STUDIO CUES
- Sit comfortably with knees lower than hips, and relax the shoulders
- Close the eyes and journey inwards
- First gently drop right ear towards right shoulder without lifting the shoulder, repeat on the left side
- Second turn and look over the right shoulder, repeat on the left side
- Thirdly, pull the chin back and then push it forward
- Lastly, come back to a neutral head position

BENEFITS

- Reduce severity of a headache
- Relax the jaw muscles
- Improve posture and release tightness from excess screen time

MODIFICATIONS

- Be careful not to drop the chin down, keep the eye gaze straight ahead
- Practice these stretches seated on a chair

PARTNER WITH:
ALL POSES

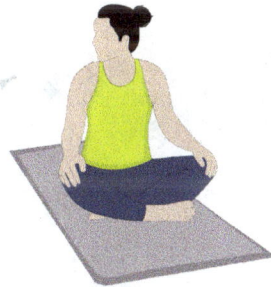

Neck Releases

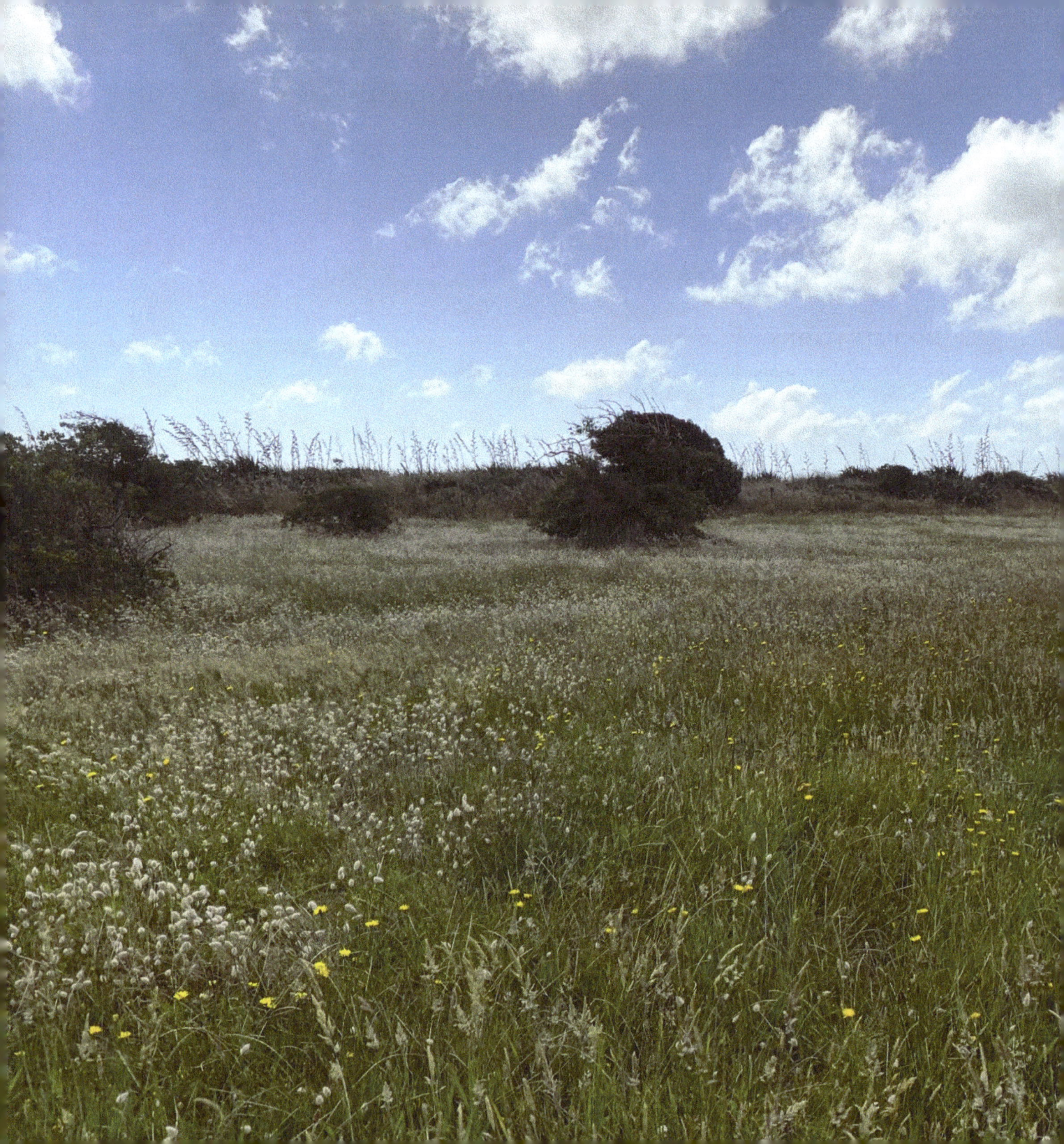

Deepening your YOGA practice

Congratulations! You have taken yourself on a journey of transformation.

Thank you for trusting me to guide you through this yoga program.

At the beginning of this book I mentioned the ability of a consistent yoga practice to help reduce pain, improve sleep, provide mental clarity and develop resilience. These were lofty goals, and I trust you are seeing the changes within yourself, sparking a desire to continue exploring yoga for your health and wellbeing.

The true power of yoga though is the conversation you are now regularly having with yourself on the mat. I invite you to take all of life's issues onto that yoga mat and work the puzzle in a deeper way. That means going beyond the physical; acknowledging when you are feeling tired and disconnected. overwhelmed with emotion (good or bad), have an upset digestive system, hormonal imbalance, or just plain confused about life's direction. Sit in the various yoga poses with the intention to release and heal, trusting your body to guide you into the next steps. In this way you will strengthen your own sense of inner guidance.

If you are interested to know more about how you can continue to transform your life then check out some of the other programs we have available. The companion to this yoga program is the 30 day Yoga Stretch Challenge, available to download at the website 35daydetox.com. Now that you are moving more it will become instinctive to stretch out any tension before it has a chance to settle and become chronic.

Eventually we all come to the realisation that to improve our physical fitness and yoga experience there is a need to change other factors such as food habits and stress levels. The 35 Day Detox Challenge was created to support this next step. As the saying go "seek and you will find".

Working with Injury and Trauma

Here are a few combinations of poses I have used in the yoga studio for specific desired outcomes. Most can be done in less than 10 minutes!   First let me repeat the proviso - please check with your medical practitioner first - your body is unique with a its own set of factors to consider.

RELIEVING SCIATICA PAIN

- A simple flow of **Mountain** to **Forward Fold** to **Half Lift** to **Forward Fold** to **Mountain** can be an effective morning practice. Follow the "one breath one movement" gentle yoga flow, making the movements small to start with. Stay out of the pain-point. Repeat a few times and then come to stillness with hands to heart. Press the feet down to the mat, tuck the tailbone under to lengthen through the spine, press the palms together, close the eyes, and take a few deep clearing breaths in through the nose and out through the mouth.
- In the evening, stretches such as **Butterfly** and **Head Beyond Knee** can offer relief.

STRENGTHENING THE KNEES

- Practice these standing poses regularly for increased stability - **Mountain** (especially with the added challenge of rising onto the toes), **Pyramid** and **Eagle**. Use the support of the foot partially on the floor to maintain good form.
- Take time to build the surrounding muscles with poses that strengthen - e.g. **Bridge** (hamstrings), **Low Lunge** (quads and calves).
- Avoid poses that create a twisting of the leg (**Triangle**, **Kneeling Hip Releases**), or bending the knee beyond 90 degrees (**Reclining Half Hero**).

STRENGTHENING THE HIPS

- All the single leg standing poses are helpful, ensuring the body is in alignment - shoulder over hip over knee over ankle - practice **Tree** and **Extended One Leg** regularly.
- Standing poses such as **Pyramid** and **Half Lift** strengthen by holding the upper body prone (90 degrees).
- On the mat **Kneeling Superman**, **Forearm Plank** and **Locust** are great for improving the hip and lower back strength. **Boat** can help with lower abdominal strength.

LOWER BACK RELIEF

- To recover and strengthen the back muscles initially spend time in **Tabletop** pose with good form. Next gently add the **Kneeling Superman.**
- Ensure there is good core strength before moving on to dynamic sequences. Longer holds in **Plank** and/or **Forearm Plank** will work all the muscles. Ensure the breathing is even and the neck muscles are relaxed.
- After the strengthening, ensure you stretch with **Extended Child's Pose** and **Head Beyond Knee**. Being mindful to engage the core (belly button to spine) to stabilise the area.

IMPROVING SHOULDER MOBILITY

- Begin with **Cat Cow** to create some movement and warmth, then the **Thread the Needle** variation that starts in **Tabletop** and gently slides the arm through. Exhale as the arm goes through and inhale as you return to **Tabletop.**
- Use the **Eagle** variation that stretches the arms wide, then forward with palms together, elbows bend and hands come back towards to the face, and last stretches out again. Stay within the range of motion that is not causing any pain response.
- Build strength with **Plank** or **Modified Plank**. Once strength is returned **Sage Variation** is a great stretch for the shoulder.
- Keep the arm low with the hand on hip in poses such as **Twisted Lunge**, **Triangle** to reduce the pressure on the shoulder.

DIGESTIVE ISSUES

- A powerful morning digestive routine would be : Start with a **Twisting Warmup**, follow with **Mountain** (onto toes if possible), one breath one movement **Standing Side Stretches**. Come down to the mat for **Cobra** with a twist, finish with the **Seated Half Spinal Twist** and **Neck Releases**.
- For a more dynamic digestive routine load the Sun Salutation Sequence with different combinations of poses each round. e.g. Round One add a hold in **Plank** plus include a twist to the **Cobra.** Round Two add **Wild Thing** after **Downdog**. Round Three add **TwistedLunge** after **Downdog**.
- In the evening practice a seated **Forward Fold**, followed by **Reclining Half Hero** and **Bridge**. Complete the sequence with **Happy Baby** and **Reclined Spinal Twist**, resting lying on your back with elbows on the floor and hands on the stomach.

REPRODUCTIVE ISSUES

- Start low to the ground, taking the time to gently stimulate the reproductive organs. Begin in **Extended Child's Pose,** feeling the gentle massaging effect of the breath's ability to move abdominal area against the upper thighs. Lift up to **Downdog** taking the opportunity to stretch down the backs of the legs. Walk hands to feet and come into **Forward Fold**, pause at **Half Lift** before placing hands to floor and stepping the right leg forward for **Low Lunge**, to **TwistedLunge**. Step back to **Downdog** and repeat for the left side.

RELIEF FROM MENOPAUSE SYMPTOMS

- The cooling effect of Hissing (Sitkari) breath can help. Place tongue on the roof of the mouth and breathe out through the mouth slowly with a hissing sound. Repeat a few times. The inhale is done through the nose.
- Gentle movement with **Cat Cow** can provide joint relief and an overall sense of wellbeing.
- Although it is tempting to curl up in a ball, the best antidote is to gently stretch out the reproductive organs. This will stimulate blood supply and movement can release tension.
- Start the day with poses such as **Mountain**, **Standing Side Stretches** and **Triangle**.
- In the evening try poses such as **Locust, Bridge, Reclining Half Hero,** and **Happy Baby.**

BALANCING HORMONES

- Consider these chemical messengers need clear pathways to function well. All yoga is working at some level to improve the body's functions.
- Spend time in the evening nurturing yourself and preparing for a good night's sleep. Start with a **Seated Half Spinal Twist**, pause and reset in the seated **Half Lift** then move to **Butterfly** followed by **Head Beyond Knee**. Lie on your back for **Happy Baby** and a reclined version of the **Kneeling Hip Releases**. Finish with the **Relaxation Meditation.**

STIMULATE THE LYMPHATIC SYSTEM

- Target the major lymph nodes around the armpits and groin with plenty of dynamic movement. The **Twisting Warmup** and **Sun Salutation** sequence are great daily practices. Add **Standing Side Stretches**, **Twisted Lunge** and **Wild Thing** to the sequence to build blood and lymph flow.
- Spend time in the **Forward Fold** with hands to elbows. At night practice **Half Lift** with legs up the wall.

STRESS RELIEF

- A lovely time to do the **Relaxation Meditation** is even before you get out of bed in the morning. Take a few minutes to connect mind to body and set up your personal priorities.
- Each morning aim to release tension from the joints and stimulate the lymphatic system. Start with **Extended Child's Pose with Side Stretches**, next mindfully work through the **Wrist Releases.** Create movement through the spine with **Cat Cow**, stretch forward to **Puppy** ensure the forehead is resting on the floor. Next perform the **Kneeling Hip Releases**, noticing the circular motion around the digestive and reproductive organs. Come onto the knees for **Gate** to activate all the energy lines and improve vitality. Last sit comfortably and do the **Neck Releases.**
- In the evening spend time in **Reclined Butterfly** and **Snow Angel**.
- Some times a strong pose is needed to break a pattern. Warmup with the Sun Salutation sequence then practice **Eagle**, **Tiger** or **Wild Thing.** The challenge of maintaining the position is all-consuming and the relief afterwards is a circuit-breaker to the stress response.

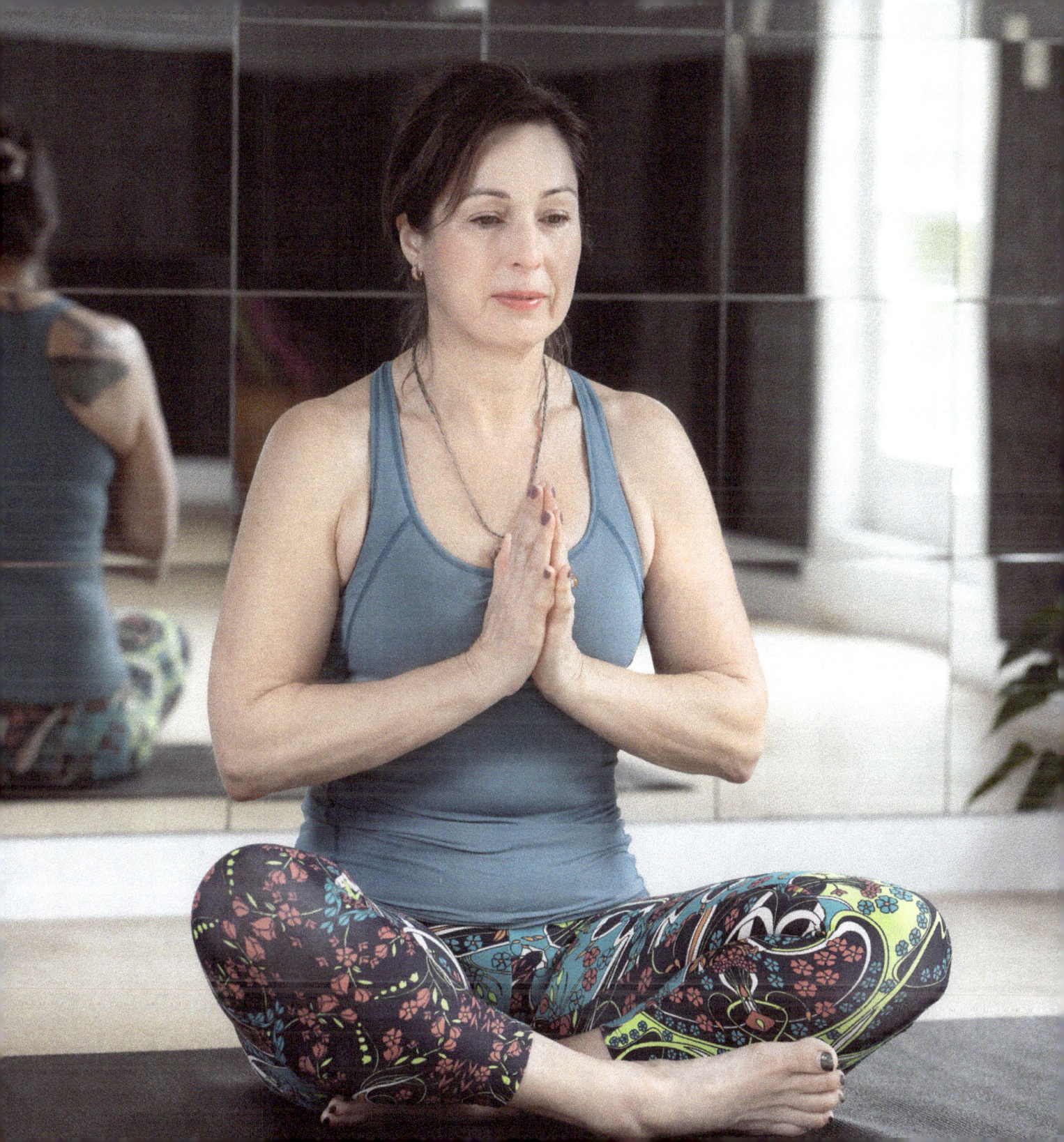

INDEX OF YOGA POSES

ABOUT THE AUTHOR

Suz Stokes lives in Raumati South, on the Kapiti Coast, New Zealand with her two dogs, Beau and Jojo. She is the founder of 35 Day Detox Ltd, a health and wellbeing company. The company provides online programs based on the principles of yoga, astrology, numerology, feng shui, healthy whole food recipes and physical fitness.

Since 2014 she was been operating a yoga studio, welcoming private clients to learn about the benefits of yoga to improve their lives. She also has a regular schedule of group classes and workshops - creating a community of individuals that priortise their own health and wellbeing through the practice of yoga.

Suz is the author of two books. The 2014 recipe book - "35 Day Detox, Manifesting Change", and a her own story "The Physical Manifestation of Self, High Heels to Yoga Pants, with a side of IRONMAN" published in 2022.